The Brain Science behind Aging and Forgetting

Unveiling the Neuroscience of Forgetfulness in Lost Memories

Peter Kattan

Petra Books
www.PetraBooks.com

The Brain Science behind Aging and Forgetting
Unveiling the Neuroscience of Forgetfulness in Lost
Memories

Preface

In an era where life expectancy is on the rise and populations are aging, understanding the intricacies of brain health becomes paramount. This book embarks on a journey through the labyrinth of the aging mind, exploring the enigmatic realm of memory, the resilience of neuroplasticity, and the profound impact of lifestyle choices on cognitive longevity.

The genesis of this work stems from a recognition of the pervasive yet often misunderstood challenges associated with aging and forgetting. Through a comprehensive examination of the latest findings in brain science, we aim to illuminate the path toward a better understanding of the aging brain and offer actionable insights for maintaining cognitive vitality.

In our exploration, we traverse the landscape of the aging brain, delving into its structural and functional transformations, deciphering the mechanisms of memory and forgetting, and uncovering the remarkable adaptability encapsulated within the concept of neuroplasticity. Along this journey, we shine a light on the pivotal role of lifestyle factors, such as diet, exercise, sleep, and stress management, in sculpting the trajectory of cognitive aging.

Furthermore, we showcase a myriad of brain-boosting activities and delve into the profound implications of social engagement and lifelong learning on brain health. Through this holistic approach, we endeavor to empower readers to take proactive steps in safeguarding their cognitive well-being.

As we peer into the future of brain aging research, we are met with promising advancements and a beacon of hope for combating age-related cognitive decline. By distilling complex scientific insights into digestible knowledge, we aspire to equip readers with the tools and knowledge necessary to navigate the intricacies of brain aging with confidence and resilience.

This book is not merely a compilation of scientific discoveries; it is a call to action, urging readers to prioritize brain health and aging in their lives. As we embark on this journey together, let us embrace the profound significance of understanding the brain science behind aging and forgetting, for therein lies the key to unlocking a future of cognitive vitality and well-being.

It should be noted that a large part of this book was written with the help of artificial intelligence, specifically using ChatGPT3.5.

Peter Kattan   August 2024

ISBN - 979-8-3303-2363-0

The Brain Science behind Aging and Forgetting Unveiling the Neuroscience of Forgetfulness in Lost Memories

Contents

Introduction: Overview of the book's focus on the brain science of aging and forgetting

The book's focus on the brain science of aging and forgetting is a profound exploration of the intricate workings of the human brain as it traverses the journey of aging. Aging is a natural process that affects every aspect of our being, including our cognitive functions and memory retention. By delving into the complexities of how the brain changes over time, we can unravel the mysteries of why we forget certain things as we grow older.

The brain, often referred to as the command center of the body, undergoes a series of transformations as we age. These changes can have a significant impact on our cognitive abilities, including memory, attention, and problem-solving skills. Understanding the mechanisms behind these changes is crucial for developing strategies to maintain brain health and cognitive function in later years.

Memory and forgetting are two sides of the same coin when it comes to aging. Memory is the process by which the brain encodes, stores, and retrieves information, while forgetting is the inability to recall certain memories or pieces of information. As we age, our memory abilities may decline due to various factors, such as changes in brain structure, neurotransmitter levels, and blood flow to the brain.

One of the key topics to be covered in this book is the impact of aging on brain structure and function. As we grow older, the brain undergoes structural changes, including shrinkage of certain regions and alterations in neural connectivity. These changes can affect cognitive functions such as memory, attention, and decision-making. By understanding how the aging brain differs from its younger counterpart, we can better appreciate the challenges and opportunities that come with aging.

Another important topic to be explored is the concept of neuroplasticity and its role in aging. Neuroplasticity refers to the brain's ability to reorganize itself by forming new neural connections in response to learning and experience. Despite the changes that occur in the aging brain, neuroplasticity allows for continued growth and adaptation throughout life. By engaging in activities that promote neuroplasticity, such as learning new skills or engaging in cognitive exercises, older adults can enhance their brain function and potentially offset some age-related cognitive decline.

Lifestyle factors also play a significant role in brain health and aging. Diet, exercise, sleep, and stress management can all impact cognitive function and memory retention. A healthy lifestyle that includes a balanced diet, regular physical activity, sufficient sleep, and effective stress management can support brain health and reduce the risk of cognitive decline as we age. By adopting healthy habits and making lifestyle changes, individuals can optimize their brain function and overall well-being in later years.

In addition to lifestyle factors, engaging in brain-boosting activities can also have a positive impact on cognitive function in older adults. Cognitive exercises, mental challenges, social engagement, and lifelong learning can all help stimulate the brain and promote cognitive vitality. By staying mentally active and socially connected, older adults can maintain cognitive function and potentially reduce the risk of age-related memory problems.

The future of brain aging research holds promise for uncovering new insights into the mechanisms of cognitive decline and memory loss in older adults. Ongoing research efforts are focused on identifying biomarkers of brain aging, developing interventions to support cognitive function in later years, and exploring innovative treatments for age-related cognitive disorders. By staying informed about the latest advancements in brain aging research, we can gain a better understanding of how to promote brain health and cognitive resilience as we age.

The brain science behind aging and forgetting is a multifaceted field that offers valuable insights into the complexities of cognitive function and memory retention in later years. By exploring the impact of aging on the brain, understanding the mechanisms of memory and forgetting, and embracing lifestyle factors that support brain health, we can empower ourselves to age gracefully and maintain optimal cognitive function throughout life. Through a comprehensive examination of key topics in brain science, this book aims to equip readers with the knowledge and strategies needed to navigate the challenges and opportunities of aging with resilience and grace.

Chapter I. The Aging Brain

Overview of how the brain changes as we age

The human brain, a marvel of complexity and adaptability, undergoes significant changes as we progress through the stages of life. Aging, a natural process, brings about various transformations in the structure and function of the brain. These changes are part of the broader spectrum of neuroplasticity, the brain's ability to reorganize itself in response to environmental and internal stimuli. Understanding how the brain evolves with age is crucial for addressing cognitive health concerns and promoting well-being in older adults.

One of the most noticeable changes in the aging brain is the decline in volume and weight. Studies have shown that starting from middle age, the brain gradually loses neurons, synapses, and white matter. These structural alterations can lead to reductions in overall brain size and changes in specific regions, such as the prefrontal cortex and hippocampus, which are vital for functions like memory, attention, and decision-making.

Moreover, aging affects the brain's biochemical and molecular composition. Neurotransmitter levels, including dopamine and serotonin, may decline, impacting mood regulation and cognitive processes. Additionally, oxidative stress and inflammation increase with age, potentially contributing to neuronal damage and cognitive decline.

Functional changes also accompany the aging process. Brain activity patterns may shift, with alterations in connectivity between different regions. Older adults may exhibit differences in neural network functioning during tasks involving memory, executive function, and processing speed. These changes can manifest as cognitive challenges, such as slower information processing, decreased working memory capacity, and difficulties in multitasking.

However, it is essential to recognize that not all aspects of brain function decline with age. Some cognitive abilities, such as crystallized intelligence and emotional regulation, may remain stable or even improve over time. Furthermore, the brain demonstrates remarkable resilience and adaptive capacity in response to aging-related changes. Neuroplasticity allows the brain to rewire circuits, form new connections, and compensate for functional deficits, albeit to a certain extent.

The aging brain undergoes a series of structural, biochemical, and functional changes that impact cognitive function and overall well-being. While some decline is inevitable, interventions aimed at promoting brain health and fostering neuroplasticity can mitigate the negative effects of aging on cognitive function. By understanding the mechanisms underlying brain aging and implementing strategies to support cognitive resilience, we can enhance the quality of life for older adults and promote healthy aging for generations to come.

Various factors influence the trajectory of brain aging and the extent of cognitive decline experienced by individuals. Genetics play a significant role, with certain gene variants associated with increased susceptibility to neurodegenerative conditions like Alzheimer's disease. Lifestyle factors, including diet, physical activity, cognitive engagement, and social interaction, also exert profound effects on brain health in later life.

As individuals age, the brain's ability to adapt and respond to new challenges becomes increasingly important. Cognitive reserve, the brain's capacity to withstand neuropathological damage, plays a crucial role in determining how well individuals can cope with age-related cognitive decline. Factors such as education, occupational complexity, and engagement in mentally stimulating activities contribute to cognitive reserve and may help buffer against the effects of aging on cognitive function.

Furthermore, social connections and engagement play a significant role in promoting brain health in older adults. Social isolation and loneliness have been linked to an increased risk of cognitive decline and neurodegenerative diseases. Maintaining strong social networks, participating in social activities, and fostering meaningful relationships can have a protective effect on cognitive function and overall brain health in later life.

Physical exercise is another key component of promoting brain health and cognitive function in aging individuals. Regular physical activity has been shown to have numerous benefits for the brain, including improved blood flow, enhanced neuroplasticity, and reduced risk of cognitive decline. Aerobic exercise, in particular, has been associated with increased brain volume in areas important for memory and executive function, highlighting the importance of staying physically active as we age.

Moreover, diet and nutrition play a critical role in supporting brain health and cognitive function in older adults. A diet rich in antioxidants, omega-3 fatty acids, and vitamins has been linked to better cognitive performance and a reduced risk of cognitive decline. Consuming a variety of fruits, vegetables, whole grains, and lean proteins can provide essential nutrients that support brain function and protect against age-related cognitive impairment.

As we age, it is important to prioritize mental stimulation and cognitive engagement to maintain brain health and cognitive function. Activities such as reading, puzzles, learning new skills, and engaging in intellectually challenging tasks can help preserve cognitive abilities and promote neuroplasticity in the aging brain. Continued learning and mental stimulation have been shown to have a protective effect against cognitive decline and may help maintain cognitive function in later life.

Overall, the aging process brings about changes that can impact cognitive function and overall well-being. While some degree of cognitive decline is incvitable with age, there are various strategies that individuals can adopt to promote brain health, enhance cognitive resilience, and improve their quality of life as they grow older. By making lifestyle adjustments, participating in mentally stimulating activities, nurturing social connections, and prioritizing physical exercise and nutrition, individuals can optimize their brain health and support healthy aging throughout their later years.

Furthermore, the significance of sleep cannot be overlooked when considering brain health and cognitive function in aging individuals. Adequate sleep is crucial for memory consolidation, cognitive processing, and overall brain health. Research indicates that chronic sleep deprivation can have detrimental effects on cognitive performance and may contribute to cognitive decline over time. Therefore, prioritizing good sleep hygiene and ensuring sufficient rest is essential for supporting cognitive function as individuals age.

Another important aspect to consider in the quest for optimal brain health is stress management. Chronic stress has been linked to cognitive impairment and can negatively impact brain function. Engaging in stress-reducing activities such as mindfulness meditation, yoga, or spending time in nature can help mitigate the effects of stress on the brain and promote overall cognitive well-being. By incorporating stress management techniques into their daily routine, individuals can better protect their cognitive abilities and support healthy aging.

Moreover, staying socially active and maintaining meaningful relationships can also play a significant role in preserving cognitive function as individuals age. Social interaction has been shown to stimulate the brain, enhance cognitive abilities, and reduce the risk of cognitive decline. Engaging in social activities, participating in group settings, and fostering connections with others can provide cognitive benefits and contribute to overall brain health in older age.

The journey towards maintaining brain health and cognitive function throughout the aging process involves a multifaceted approach that encompasses various aspects of lifestyle and behavior. By integrating strategies such as proper nutrition, mental stimulation, adequate sleep, stress management, and social engagement into their daily lives, individuals can proactively support their cognitive abilities, promote brain health, and enhance their overall quality of life as they age. Embracing these holistic approaches can empower individuals to age gracefully and maintain cognitive resilience well into their later years.

Furthermore, physical exercise is a crucial component of maintaining brain health and cognitive function as individuals age. Regular physical activity has been associated with improved cognitive performance, enhanced memory, and a reduced risk of cognitive decline. Exercise promotes blood flow to the brain, stimulates the release of growth factors that support brain health, and helps in the formation of new neural connections. By incorporating a mix of aerobic exercise, strength training, and flexibility exercises into their routine, individuals can support brain health and cognitive function as they age.

Closely related to physical exercise is the importance of maintaining a healthy weight and managing cardiovascular health. Research suggests that obesity, high blood pressure, and other cardiovascular risk factors can have negative effects on brain health and cognitive function. By adopting a healthy lifestyle that includes regular exercise, a balanced diet, and routine medical check-ups to monitor cardiovascular health, individuals can reduce their risk of cognitive decline and support brain health in the long term.

Additionally, engaging in activities that promote emotional well-being and mental health can also benefit cognitive function in older age. Practices such as mindfulness, relaxation techniques, and hobbies that bring joy and fulfillment can help reduce anxiety, depression, and stress, all of which can impact cognitive abilities. Prioritizing mental and emotional well-being is essential for maintaining cognitive resilience and supporting overall brain health as individuals navigate the aging process.

Lastly, staying intellectually curious and open to new experiences can further enhance cognitive function and brain health in older age. Lifelong learning, exploring new interests, and challenging oneself intellectually can help keep the brain active and engaged. By seeking out opportunities for intellectual growth and embracing new challenges, individuals can continue to stimulate their cognitive abilities, foster neuroplasticity, and promote healthy aging of the brain.

The journey towards preserving brain health and cognitive function in later years involves a comprehensive approach that encompasses various lifestyle factors and behaviors. By integrating strategies such as physical exercise, cardiovascular health management, emotional well-being practices, and intellectual stimulation into their daily lives, individuals can proactively support their cognitive abilities, promote brain health, and enhance their overall quality of life as they age. Embracing a holistic approach to brain health can empower individuals to age gracefully, maintain cognitive resilience, and continue to thrive cognitively well into their later years.

Impact of aging on brain structure and function

The aging process exerts a profound impact on the structure and function of the human brain, influencing cognitive abilities and behavior in significant ways. As individuals grow older, they experience a multitude of changes at the cellular, molecular, and systemic levels, contributing to alterations in brain structure and function. Understanding the nature and implications of these changes is essential for addressing age-related cognitive decline and promoting brain health in older adults.

Structurally, the aging brain undergoes several notable transformations. One of the most prominent changes is cortical thinning, particularly in regions associated with higher-order cognitive functions such as the prefrontal cortex. This thinning is thought to reflect neuronal loss and reductions in synaptic density, leading to declines in executive function, working memory, and attention.

Moreover, aging is associated with alterations in white matter integrity, the brain's network of myelinated axons that facilitate communication between different regions. Degenerative processes, including demyelination and axonal damage, can compromise the efficiency of neural transmission and disrupt connectivity within neural networks. These white matter changes are implicated in cognitive decline and increased vulnerability to neurodegenerative diseases such as Alzheimer's and Parkinson's.

Functional changes in the aging brain are equally consequential. Neuroimaging studies have revealed age-related differences in patterns of brain activation during cognitive tasks, indicating shifts in neural recruitment and network dynamics. Older adults often exhibit reduced neural efficiency and compensatory recruitment of additional brain regions to maintain performance on cognitive tasks, a phenomenon known as the compensation-related utilization of neural circuits hypothesis (CRUNCH).

Furthermore, aging affects neurotransmitter systems, such as dopamine, acetylcholine, and serotonin, which play critical roles in modulating cognitive function and behavior. Changes in neurotransmitter levels and receptor sensitivity contribute to alterations in mood, motivation, and cognitive processes, potentially exacerbating age-related cognitive decline.

The impact of aging on brain structure and function is influenced by a myriad of factors, including genetic predisposition, lifestyle choices, and environmental exposures. While genetic factors contribute to individual differences in susceptibility to age-related cognitive decline and neurodegenerative diseases, lifestyle interventions such as physical exercise, cognitive stimulation, and social engagement can promote brain health and mitigate the negative effects of aging on cognitive function.

Aging exerts a multifaceted impact on the structure and function of the brain, leading to alterations in cognition, behavior, and overall well-being. By elucidating the mechanisms underlying age-related changes in the brain and implementing targeted interventions, we can enhance cognitive resilience and promote healthy aging across the lifespan.

Apart from the mentioned structural and functional changes, aging also affects neuroplasticity, the brain's ability to adapt and reorganize in response to experiences and environmental stimuli. While neuroplasticity decreases with age, interventions like cognitive training and mindfulness practices can enhance plasticity and support cognitive function in older adults.

Additionally, aging leads to alterations in inflammatory processes, oxidative stress, and mitochondrial function, which can contribute to neuronal damage and cognitive decline. Chronic inflammation and oxidative stress are involved in the development of neurodegenerative diseases, emphasizing the importance of lifestyle interventions that reduce inflammation and boost antioxidant defenses.

Aging is also linked to changes in the blood-brain barrier, the protective barrier regulating substance passage between the bloodstream and the brain. Blood-brain barrier disruption can increase permeability, allowing harmful substances to enter the brain and contribute to neuro inflammation and neuronal dysfunction.

Furthermore, the aging process is associated with changes in synaptic plasticity, the ability of neurons to form and reorganize connections in response to experiences. Age-related alterations in synaptic plasticity can impact learning and memory processes, contributing to cognitive decline in older adults. Strategies that promote synaptic plasticity, such as engaging in challenging cognitive tasks, learning new skills, and maintaining social interactions, can help support cognitive function and mitigate the effects of aging on brain plasticity.

In addition to synaptic plasticity, the aging brain is also influenced by changes in neuroinflammation, oxidative stress, and mitochondrial function. Chronic inflammation and oxidative stress can damage neurons and impair cognitive function, while mitochondrial dysfunction can disrupt energy production in brain cells. Lifestyle interventions that reduce inflammation, enhance antioxidant defenses, and support mitochondrial health, such as a balanced diet rich in antioxidants and regular exercise, can help protect the aging brain from these detrimental processes.

Moreover, aging is associated with alterations in the gut-brain axis, the bidirectional communication system between the gastrointestinal tract and the brain. Changes in gut microbiota composition and function can influence brain health and cognitive function through the production of neurotransmitters, immune modulation, and the regulation of inflammation. Maintaining a healthy gut microbiome through a diverse diet, probiotics, and prebiotics can positively impact brain health and cognitive function in older adults.

Furthermore, the impact of aging on the brain extends to the regulation of stress hormones, such as cortisol, which plays a role in the body's response to stress. Dysregulation of the stress response system in older adults can have negative effects on brain health and cognitive function, leading to increased vulnerability to cognitive decline and mood disorders. Stress management techniques, such as mindfulness, meditation, relaxation exercises, and regular physical activity, can help regulate stress hormone levels and support brain health in aging individuals.

Additionally, age-related changes in the blood-brain barrier can affect the brain's ability to maintain a stable internal environment and protect against harmful substances. Disruption of the blood-brain barrier integrity can lead to increased permeability, allowing toxins and inflammatory molecules to enter the brain and contribute to neuroinflammation and neuronal dysfunction. Protecting the integrity of the blood-brain barrier through lifestyle factors like a healthy diet, adequate hydration, and regular exercise is crucial for maintaining brain health and cognitive function in older age.

The aging brain undergoes a multitude of changes that impact its structure, function, and overall health. By understanding the complex interplay of factors involved in brain aging and implementing a holistic approach that addresses synaptic plasticity, neuroinflammation, gut-brain axis function, stress regulation, and blood-brain barrier integrity, individuals can support cognitive function, promote brain health, and enhance overall well-being as they age. Continued research into the mechanisms of brain aging and the development of targeted interventions will be essential for optimizing cognitive resilience and quality of life in older adults.

Moreover, aging is also associated with alterations in sleep patterns and circadian rhythms, which play a crucial role in cognitive function and overall brain health. Disrupted sleep and irregular circadian rhythms can impair memory consolidation, attention, and cognitive performance, contributing to age-related cognitive decline. Strategies to promote healthy sleep habits and maintain a regular sleep-wake cycle, such as creating a relaxing bedtime routine, limiting screen time before bed, and optimizing the sleep environment, can support cognitive function and brain health in older adults.

Furthermore, age-related changes in hormonal regulation, such as a decline in sex hormones like estrogen and testosterone, can impact brain function and cognition. Hormonal fluctuations in aging individuals can affect mood, memory, and cognitive processes, leading to symptoms like mood swings, fatigue, and cognitive impairment. Hormone replacement therapy under medical supervision and lifestyle modifications that support hormonal balance, such as regular exercise and stress management, can help mitigate the effects of hormonal changes on brain health and cognitive function in older adults.

Additionally, aging is linked to alterations in neurovascular coupling, the mechanism that ensures adequate blood flow to active brain regions during cognitive tasks. Impaired neurovascular coupling in older adults can lead to reduced oxygen and nutrient delivery to brain cells, affecting cognitive performance and increasing the risk of cognitive decline. Physical activity, cardiovascular fitness, and a healthy diet rich in nutrients that support vascular health can enhance neurovascular coupling and promote optimal brain function in aging individuals.

Moreover, age-related changes in neurogenesis, the process of generating new neurons in the brain, can impact cognitive function and brain plasticity. Reduced neurogenesis in aging individuals may contribute to cognitive decline and impair the brain's ability to adapt and respond to environmental stimuli. Lifestyle factors that support neurogenesis, such as regular aerobic exercise, a diet rich in omega-3 fatty acids, and cognitive stimulation, can help maintain cognitive function and support brain plasticity in older age.

Furthermore, aging is associated with alterations in the brain's immune response, known as immunosenescence, which can impact neuroinflammation and neuronal health. Dysregulation of the immune system in older adults can lead to chronic low-grade inflammation in the brain, contributing to cognitive decline and neurodegenerative diseases. Strategies that support immune function, such as a balanced diet, regular exercise, and stress reduction techniques, can help modulate neuroinflammation and promote brain health in aging individuals.

The aging brain undergoes a complex interplay of changes that affect its structure, function, and overall health. By addressing various aspects of brain aging, including sleep patterns, hormonal regulation, neurovascular coupling, neurogenesis, and immune function, individuals can support cognitive resilience, promote brain health, and enhance quality of life as they age. Continued research into the mechanisms of brain aging and the development of personalized interventions will be crucial for optimizing cognitive function and well-being in older adults.

Factors that contribute to cognitive decline in older adults

Cognitive decline is a common and often feared aspect of aging, affecting millions of older adults worldwide. While some degree of cognitive changes is considered a normal part of aging, significant decline can impair daily functioning and diminish quality of life. Understanding the factors that contribute to cognitive decline in older adults is essential for developing effective strategies to promote brain health and preserve cognitive function as individuals age.

One of the primary contributors to cognitive decline in older adults is neurodegenerative diseases, such as Alzheimer's disease, Parkinson's disease, and vascular dementia. These conditions are characterized by progressive degeneration of brain tissue, leading to impairments in memory, attention, language, and executive function. Genetic factors, including mutations in genes such as APOE4, increase the risk of developing neurodegenerative diseases and accelerating cognitive decline.

In addition to neurodegenerative processes, age-related changes in brain structure and function play a significant role in cognitive decline. As individuals grow older, they experience reductions in gray matter volume, alterations in white matter integrity, and changes in neurotransmitter systems, all of which can contribute to declines in cognitive abilities. Structural changes in the brain, such as cortical thinning and hippocampal atrophy, are particularly associated with impairments in memory and executive function.

Furthermore, vascular risk factors, such as hypertension, diabetes, and obesity, increase the likelihood of cognitive decline in older adults. These conditions can lead to cerebral small vessel disease, stroke, and microvascular pathology, impairing blood flow to the brain and compromising neural function. Chronic inflammation, oxidative stress, and metabolic dysfunction associated with vascular risk factors contribute to neuronal damage and cognitive impairment.

Lifestyle factors also play a crucial role in cognitive decline and brain health in older adults. Sedentary behavior, poor diet, smoking, and excessive alcohol consumption are associated with increased risk of cognitive decline and dementia. Conversely, engaging in regular physical activity, following a balanced diet rich in fruits, vegetables, and omega-3 fatty acids, and maintaining social and cognitive engagement can help preserve cognitive function and reduce the risk of age-related cognitive decline.

Psychosocial factors, such as education, socioeconomic status, and social support, also influence cognitive aging trajectories.

Cognitive decline is a complex issue affecting many elderly individuals globally. While some cognitive changes are expected with age, significant decline can be daunting for individuals and their families. It is crucial to understand the various factors contributing to cognitive decline in older adults to develop strategies for promoting brain health and preserving cognitive function in later life.

Neurodegenerative diseases, such as Alzheimer's, Parkinson's, and vascular dementia, are major contributors to cognitive decline. Genetic predispositions, like APOE4 mutations, can heighten susceptibility to these diseases, hastening cognitive decline.

Age-related changes in brain structure and function also play a significant role in cognitive decline. As individuals age, changes in gray matter volume, white matter integrity, and neurotransmitter systems collectively contribute to declines in cognitive abilities. Structural brain transformations, such as cortical thinning and hippocampal atrophy, are particularly implicated in memory impairments and executive function deficits in the elderly.

Vascular risk factors, including hypertension, diabetes, and obesity, exacerbate cognitive decline by fostering the development of cerebral small vessel disease and compromising neural function. Lifestyle choices, such as physical activity and a balanced diet, can impact cognitive health and resilience. Conversely, sedentary lifestyles, unhealthy dietary habits, and excessive alcohol consumption are linked to heightened risks of cognitive decline and dementia.

Psychosocial determinants, including educational attainment, socioeconomic status, and social support networks, also influence cognitive aging. Higher education levels and strong social support systems can potentially shield individuals from the effects of cognitive decline.

Cognitive decline in older adults is influenced by various factors. By understanding and addressing these contributors, holistic strategies can be developed to promote brain health, preserve cognitive function, and enhance the quality of life for aging individuals. As research in neuroscience and gerontology advances, there is increasing recognition of the multifaceted nature of cognitive decline and the importance of adopting a comprehensive approach to mitigate its impact. Interventions targeting modifiable risk factors, such as promoting cardiovascular health through regular exercise and healthy eating, have shown promise in reducing the risk of cognitive impairment. Additionally, cognitive training programs and social engagement initiatives have been instrumental in enhancing cognitive reserve and fostering resilience against age-related cognitive decline. Collaborative efforts between healthcare providers, researchers, policymakers, and community organizations are essential in developing integrated strategies that address the diverse determinants of cognitive aging and support healthy brain aging for older adults worldwide.

Cognitive decline in older adults is a multifaceted issue influenced by a variety of factors that interact in complex ways. Beyond neurodegenerative diseases, age-related changes in brain structure and function, vascular risk factors, lifestyle choices, and psychosocial determinants all contribute to the trajectory of cognitive aging.

In addition to genetic predispositions like APOE4 mutations, environmental factors also play a significant role in cognitive decline. Chronic stress, exposure to environmental toxins, and lack of mental stimulation can all contribute to cognitive impairment in older adults. Understanding the interplay between genetic and environmental factors is crucial for developing personalized interventions to mitigate cognitive decline.

Age-related changes in neurotransmitter systems, such as reductions in dopamine and acetylcholine levels, can also impact cognitive function in older adults. These changes can affect attention, memory, and executive function, highlighting the importance of maintaining a healthy brain environment through lifestyle choices and targeted interventions.

Vascular risk factors not only contribute to cognitive decline but also increase the risk of stroke and other cerebrovascular events that can further impair cognitive function. Managing conditions like hypertension and diabetes through medication, lifestyle modifications, and regular monitoring is essential for preserving brain health and reducing the risk of cognitive impairment in older adults.

Lifestyle factors continue to be a critical determinant of cognitive health in aging populations. Engaging in regular physical activity, maintaining a balanced diet, staying socially and cognitively active, and avoiding harmful substances like tobacco and excessive alcohol can all help promote brain health and reduce the risk of cognitive decline.

Psychosocial factors, such as educational attainment, socioeconomic status, and social support networks, also play a crucial role in cognitive aging. Access to education, financial resources, and strong social connections can buffer against the effects of cognitive decline and support healthy brain aging in older adults.

Addressing cognitive decline in older adults requires a comprehensive approach that considers the diverse factors influencing cognitive aging. By integrating insights from genetics, neuroscience, gerontology, and public health, tailored interventions can be developed to promote brain health, preserve cognitive function, and enhance the overall quality of life for aging individuals. Collaborative efforts across disciplines and sectors are essential for advancing our understanding of cognitive decline and implementing effective strategies to support healthy brain aging worldwide.

As research in neuroscience and gerontology progresses, new insights into cognitive decline in older adults continue to emerge. Advances in neuroimaging techniques allow for a deeper understanding of how structural and functional brain changes contribute to cognitive impairment. Studying the relationships between brain regions, neural networks, and cognitive functions can provide valuable information for developing targeted interventions to preserve cognitive function in aging individuals.

Emerging evidence suggests that interventions focusing on cognitive training, mindfulness practices, and social engagement can enhance cognitive reserve and promote resilience against age-related cognitive decline. By stimulating neural plasticity and promoting neuroprotective mechanisms, these interventions have the potential to slow down cognitive decline and improve overall brain health in older adults.

Furthermore, the role of sleep quality and patterns in cognitive aging is gaining attention. Adequate sleep is essential for memory consolidation, cognitive processing, and overall brain function. Sleep disturbances, such as insomnia and sleep apnea, have been linked to cognitive deficits and an increased risk of neurodegenerative diseases. Addressing sleep-related issues through behavioral interventions and medical treatments can have a positive impact on cognitive health in older adults.

In addition to individual-level interventions, community-based programs and policies play a crucial role in promoting healthy brain aging. Creating age-friendly environments, implementing cognitive screening programs, and providing access to mental health services can support older adults in maintaining cognitive function and independence as they age. By fostering a culture of brain health awareness and prioritizing cognitive well-being, societies can better address the challenges associated with cognitive decline in aging populations.

Moreover, ongoing research on the gut-brain axis and the role of the microbiome in cognitive function is shedding light on the influence of gut health on brain health. Maintaining a diverse and balanced gut microbiota through a healthy diet rich in fiber and probiotics may have positive effects on cognitive function and reduce the risk of cognitive decline in older adults.

The field of cognitive aging is dynamic and evolving, with new discoveries shaping our understanding of how to promote healthy brain aging. By embracing a holistic approach that considers the intricate interplay of genetic, environmental, lifestyle, and psychosocial factors, we can develop innovative strategies to support cognitive health and well-being in older adults. Through continued collaboration and interdisciplinary research, we can work towards a future where cognitive decline is not inevitable, and older adults can age with dignity and cognitive vitality.

As the global population continues to age, the need for scalable and sustainable interventions to support healthy brain aging becomes increasingly urgent. Leveraging technology and digital health solutions can enhance access to cognitive training programs, telehealth services, and remote monitoring tools for older adults. Virtual platforms and mobile applications offer innovative ways to deliver personalized interventions and support cognitive wellness in diverse populations worldwide.

Furthermore, the role of social determinants of health in cognitive aging cannot be overlooked. Addressing disparities in access to healthcare, education, and social services is essential for promoting equitable brain health outcomes among older adults. Community organizations, advocacy groups, and policymakers must work together to create inclusive and supportive environments that prioritize cognitive health and well-being for all individuals as they age.

Incorporating principles of precision medicine into the field of cognitive aging holds promise for developing tailored interventions that target individual risk factors and genetic predispositions. By integrating genetic testing, biomarker analysis, and personalized lifestyle recommendations, healthcare providers can offer personalized strategies to optimize brain health and cognitive function in older adults.

Moreover, fostering a culture of lifelong learning and cognitive stimulation can have profound benefits for brain health across the lifespan. Encouraging intellectual curiosity, promoting engagement in challenging activities, and supporting ongoing education opportunities can help build cognitive reserve and resilience against age-related cognitive decline. Embracing a growth mindset and staying intellectually active are key components of a holistic approach to maintaining cognitive vitality in older age.

Collaboration between researchers, healthcare professionals, policymakers, and community stakeholders is crucial for advancing the field of cognitive aging and translating scientific discoveries into real-world impact. By fostering interdisciplinary partnerships and sharing knowledge across sectors, we can accelerate progress in developing effective interventions, raising awareness about cognitive health, and advocating for policies that support healthy brain aging for older adults around the globe.

The journey towards promoting healthy brain aging for older adults is multifaceted and requires a collective effort to address the diverse determinants of cognitive decline. By embracing innovation, inclusivity, personalized approaches, and lifelong learning, we can pave the way for a future where older adults can age with resilience, cognitive vitality, and dignity. Together, we can shape a world where cognitive aging is viewed not as a burden, but as an opportunity for growth, connection, and continued well-being.

Chapter II. Memory and Forgetting

Explanation of how memory works in the brain

Memory is a complex and fascinating aspect of human cognition, allowing us to store, retrieve, and utilize information acquired through our experiences. Understanding how memory works in the brain involves unraveling the intricate processes involved in encoding, consolidation, storage, and retrieval of information.

At its core, memory involves a series of neural networks and circuits distributed throughout the brain. The process begins with encoding, where sensory information is transformed into a format that can be stored in the brain. This process occurs primarily in the hippocampus, a region crucial for the formation of new memories. Encoding can occur through various mechanisms, including visual, auditory, semantic, and procedural processing.

Once information is encoded, it undergoes consolidation, a process by which newly formed memories are stabilized and integrated into long-term storage. Consolidation involves the strengthening of synaptic connections between neurons and the reorganization of neural circuits. The hippocampus plays a vital role in the initial stages of consolidation, but over time, memories become distributed across a network of brain regions, including the neocortex.

Stored memories can be retrieved through processes such as recognition, recall, and relearning. Recognition involves identifying previously encountered information when presented with relevant cues or stimuli. Recall, on the other hand, requires retrieving information from memory without external cues, often through associations with related concepts or contexts. Relearning involves reacquiring information that has been previously learned but forgotten.

Memory is not a unitary process but consists of multiple systems and types, each serving distinct functions and operating within different brain regions. The most widely recognized distinction is between short-term and long-term memory. Short-term memory, also known as working memory, temporarily holds information for immediate use and is supported by frontal and parietal brain regions. Long-term memory encompasses the storage of information over extended periods and is distributed across cortical regions.

Long-term memory can be further subdivided into explicit (declarative) and implicit (non-declarative) memory systems. Explicit memory involves the conscious recollection of facts and events and includes episodic and semantic memory. Episodic memory pertains to autobiographical events and experiences, while semantic memory encompasses general knowledge and facts. Implicit memory, on the other hand, operates unconsciously and includes procedural memory (skills and habits) and priming (enhanced identification of previously encountered stimuli).

Understanding the neural basis of memory has been greatly advanced through research utilizing techniques such as neuroimaging, electrophysiology, and lesion studies. Neuroimaging studies have identified brain regions implicated in various aspects of memory processing, including the hippocampus, prefrontal cortex, temporal lobes, and basal ganglia. Electrophysiological recordings have provided insights into the neural dynamics underlying memory formation and retrieval, while lesion studies have elucidated the roles of specific brain regions in different types of memory.

Memory is a multifaceted cognitive process supported by a distributed network of brain regions. From encoding and consolidation to storage and retrieval, the mechanisms underlying memory involve intricate interactions between neurons, synapses, and neural circuits. By unraveling the mysteries of memory formation and function, researchers continue to shed light on how the brain processes and preserves our past experiences.

As our understanding of memory deepens, researchers have also delved into the complexities of memory modulation and plasticity. Memory modulation refers to the processes by which memories can be modified or updated, often influenced by various factors such as emotion, attention, and prior experiences. For instance, emotionally charged events tend to be better remembered due to the activation of the amygdala, a brain region involved in processing emotions, which enhances memory consolidation.

Moreover, memory plasticity refers to the brain's ability to reorganize its neural circuits in response to experiences or learning. This phenomenon is crucial for adaptive behaviors and learning new skills. One remarkable example of memory plasticity is synaptic plasticity, the ability of synapses to strengthen or weaken over time in response to activity. Long-term potentiation (LTP) and long-term depression (LTD) are two forms of synaptic plasticity that play key roles in memory formation and storage.

Another fascinating aspect of memory is its susceptibility to distortion and false memories. Our memories are not immutable records of past events but are instead reconstructed and influenced by various factors, including suggestion, imagination, and social influences. This phenomenon has significant implications for eyewitness testimony and the reliability of memory in legal contexts.

Furthermore, research has highlighted the role of sleep in memory consolidation. Sleep, particularly the rapid eye movement (REM) stage, is essential for the consolidation of declarative memories, such as facts and events. During sleep, the brain processes and integrates newly acquired information, leading to enhanced memory retention. Disruptions in sleep patterns, such as insomnia or sleep deprivation, can impair memory consolidation and cognitive function.

Additionally, advances in technology have enabled researchers to explore the potential for enhancing memory through interventions such as brain stimulation and pharmacological agents. Transcranial magnetic stimulation (TMS) and transcranial direct current stimulation (tDCS) are non-invasive techniques that can modulate neural activity and have shown promise in improving memory performance. Similarly, pharmacological interventions targeting neurotransmitter systems involved in memory, such as acetylcholine and glutamate, hold potential for enhancing memory function in clinical settings.

The study of memory extends beyond individual cognition to encompass collective or cultural memory, which refers to the shared memories and narratives of a group or society. Collective memory plays a fundamental role in shaping cultural identity, social cohesion, and historical consciousness. Understanding how collective memories are formed, transmitted, and preserved can provide valuable insights into social dynamics, identity formation, and historical narratives.

Memory is a multifaceted and dynamic cognitive process that relies on a distributed network of brain regions and intricate neural mechanisms. From memory modulation and plasticity to the influence of sleep and societal factors, our understanding of memory continues to evolve, shedding light on the fundamental workings of the human mind. By unraveling the mysteries of memory, researchers aim to not only elucidate the mechanisms underlying cognition but also to develop interventions for enhancing memory function and preserving our collective heritage.

Moreover, recent research has highlighted the role of neurogenesis, the generation of new neurons, in memory processes. While traditionally believed to occur primarily during early development, neurogenesis continues to take place in specific brain regions, such as the hippocampus, throughout adulthood. This ongoing generation of neurons has been implicated in various aspects of memory, including pattern separation, the ability to distinguish between similar experiences or stimuli. Furthermore, factors such as physical exercise, environmental enrichment, and certain pharmacological agents have been shown to promote neurogenesis and enhance memory function.

In addition to understanding the mechanisms underlying memory, researchers are also exploring practical applications of memory research in areas such as education, therapy, and technology. Educational strategies informed by cognitive psychology and neuroscience principles aim to optimize learning and memory retention in academic settings. For example, techniques such as spaced repetition, interleaved practice, and retrieval practice have been shown to enhance long-term memory retention and learning efficiency. Similarly, therapeutic interventions for memory-related disorders, such as Alzheimer's disease and amnesia, are continually being refined based on insights from basic research on memory mechanisms.

Furthermore, advancements in brain-computer interfaces (BCIs) hold promise for augmenting human memory and cognitive function. BCIs are devices that enable direct communication between the brain and external devices, allowing for the recording, stimulation, or modulation of neural activity. In the context of memory, BCIs could potentially be used to bypass damaged or dysfunctional brain regions and restore memory function in individuals with neurological disorders. Additionally, research on neural prostheses and memory implants seeks to develop devices capable of enhancing memory encoding, storage, and retrieval in both clinical and non-clinical settings.

Another area of active research is the exploration of evolutionary perspectives on memory. Evolutionary psychologists seek to understand how memory systems have evolved over time to serve adaptive functions in ancestral environments. For example, the ability to remember the location of food sources or potential threats would have conferred survival advantages to early humans. By studying memory mechanisms across species and tracing their evolutionary origins, researchers aim to uncover the fundamental principles underlying memory function and its adaptive significance.

Moreover, interdisciplinary approaches that integrate insights from neuroscience, psychology, computer science, and other fields hold promise for advancing our understanding of memory. Collaborative efforts between researchers from diverse disciplines can lead to innovative methodologies, theoretical frameworks, and technological solutions for tackling complex questions about memory. By fostering collaboration and interdisciplinary dialogue, the field of memory research can continue to make significant strides towards unraveling the mysteries of the human mind and developing practical applications for enhancing cognitive function and well-being.

Furthermore, the study of memory intersects with various other domains of cognitive science, including perception, attention, and language. For instance, research on the relationship between attention and memory has revealed how selective attention influences what information gets encoded into memory and subsequently retrieved. Similarly, investigations into the role of language in memory have shown how linguistic factors, such as the organization of information in sentences or narratives, can affect memory performance and recall.

Additionally, cultural and societal factors shape the ways in which memories are constructed, shared, and preserved. Collective memory studies examine how groups, communities, and societies remember and commemorate significant events, shaping cultural identities and collective narratives. This interdisciplinary field draws on insights from history, sociology, anthropology, and psychology to understand how memories are transmitted across generations, perpetuated through rituals and traditions, and contested or revised over time.

Moreover, the advent of big data and computational approaches has revolutionized the study of memory by enabling the analysis of large-scale datasets and complex network dynamics. Computational models of memory aim to simulate and elucidate the underlying mechanisms of memory processes, providing insights that complement experimental findings. These models can simulate neural networks, synaptic plasticity, and learning algorithms to understand how memories are encoded, consolidated, and retrieved in the brain.

Furthermore, research on memory extends beyond individual cognition to explore social and collaborative aspects of remembering. Studies on collaborative memory investigate how individuals collectively encode, store, and retrieve information in social contexts, such as group discussions or collaborative problem-solving tasks. This research sheds light on the interplay between individual and collective memory processes, highlighting the role of social interaction, communication, and shared experiences in shaping our memories.

In the realm of artificial intelligence (AI), efforts to develop memory systems for machines have led to significant advances in fields such as natural language processing, robotics, and autonomous systems. Memory-augmented neural networks, inspired by human memory systems, incorporate mechanisms for storing and retrieving information over time, enabling machines to learn from past experiences and make contextually informed decisions. These AI systems hold promise for applications in fields such as personalized recommendation systems, autonomous navigation, and human-robot interaction.

Moreover, interdisciplinary collaborations between memory researchers and practitioners in fields such as education, healthcare, and technology are essential for translating scientific discoveries into real-world applications. Educational interventions informed by memory research can improve teaching strategies, curriculum design, and student learning outcomes. Similarly, memory-enhancing technologies and interventions have the potential to improve quality of life for individuals with memory-related disorders, such as dementia or traumatic brain injury.

The study of memory encompasses a diverse range of disciplines, methodologies, and applications, reflecting its central importance to human cognition and society. From understanding the neural mechanisms underlying memory processes to exploring the cultural, social, and computational dimensions of memory, researchers continue to uncover new insights and develop innovative approaches for harnessing the power of memory in both individual and collective contexts. By integrating knowledge from multiple disciplines and fostering interdisciplinary collaborations, the field of memory research remains at the forefront of scientific inquiry and innovation, with profound implications for our understanding of the human mind and the development of technologies to enhance memory function and well-being.

Types of memory and how they are affected by aging

Memory is a fundamental aspect of human cognition, encompassing a variety of systems and processes that allow us to store and retrieve information. As individuals age, changes in the brain can affect different types of memory, leading to variations in cognitive function and performance. Understanding the types of memory and how they are influenced by aging is crucial for addressing age-related cognitive decline and preserving cognitive function in older adults.

One of the most well-known distinctions in memory is between short-term and long-term memory. Short-term memory, also referred to as working memory, involves the temporary storage and manipulation of information for immediate use. Tasks such as remembering a phone number or following directions rely on the functionality of working memory. Aging can impact working memory capacity, with older adults typically exhibiting declines in their ability to maintain and manipulate information over short time spans.

Long-term memory encompasses the storage of information over extended periods, ranging from minutes to years. This type of memory can be further divided into explicit (declarative) and implicit (non-declarative) memory systems. Explicit memory involves the conscious recollection of facts and events and includes episodic and semantic memory. Episodic memory refers to autobiographical events and experiences, while semantic memory encompasses general knowledge and facts. Aging tends to affect episodic memory more significantly than semantic memory, with older adults experiencing difficulties in recalling specific details of past events.

Implicit memory operates unconsciously and includes procedural memory and priming. Procedural memory involves the learning and retention of skills and habits, such as riding a bike or tying shoelaces. Priming refers to the facilitated processing of stimuli as a result of prior exposure, leading to enhanced identification or production of related stimuli. While implicit memory remains relatively preserved with age, older adults may exhibit subtle declines in procedural learning and motor skill acquisition.

Another distinction in memory is between prospective and retrospective memory. Prospective memory involves remembering to perform intended actions in the future, such as attending appointments or taking medication. Retrospective memory, on the other hand, pertains to the recall of past events and information. Aging can affect both prospective and retrospective memory, with older adults experiencing difficulties in remembering future intentions and retrieving specific details from their past.

Aging-related changes in the brain, including alterations in neural structure and function, contribute to variations in memory performance. Structural changes, such as reductions in gray matter volume and alterations in white matter integrity, can impact the efficiency of neural processing and communication. Functional changes in brain networks involved in memory encoding, consolidation, and retrieval may lead to declines in cognitive abilities associated with aging.

Moreover, age-related conditions such as Alzheimer's disease and other forms of dementia can exacerbate memory problems in older adults. These neurodegenerative diseases are characterized by progressive cognitive decline and memory impairment, ultimately affecting multiple aspects of cognitive function and daily functioning.

Memory encompasses a variety of systems and processes that allow us to store and retrieve information. Aging can affect different types of memory, leading to variations in cognitive function and performance. By understanding the types of memory and how they are influenced by aging, researchers and clinicians can develop targeted interventions to preserve cognitive function and enhance quality of life in older adults.

Memory, a cornerstone of human cognition, comprises an array of mechanisms facilitating the storage and retrieval of information. As individuals progress through life, alterations in the brain may impact various facets of memory, consequently influencing cognitive function and performance. The comprehension of these memory types and their susceptibility to aging is pivotal in combatting age-related cognitive decline and upholding cognitive vitality among the elderly.

Alterations in the aging brain, encompassing changes in neural structure and functionality, contribute to variances in memory performance. Structural modifications, including reductions in gray matter volume and alterations in white matter integrity, can impact neural processing efficiency and communication. Functional alterations in brain networks implicated in memory encoding, consolidation, and retrieval may precipitate declines in cognitive capacities associated with aging.

Furthermore, age-related conditions such as Alzheimer's disease and various forms of dementia can exacerbate memory issues in older populations. These neurodegenerative ailments are typified by progressive cognitive deterioration and memory impairment, ultimately affecting numerous facets of cognitive function and daily life.

Memory constitutes a diverse array of systems and processes facilitating information storage and retrieval. Aging can influence different memory types, resulting in variations in cognitive function and performance. By comprehending these memory distinctions and their susceptibility to aging, researchers and healthcare professionals can devise targeted interventions aimed at preserving cognitive function and augmenting quality of life among older individuals.

Further investigation into the intricate relationship between memory and aging unveils a complex interplay of factors contributing to cognitive decline in older individuals. Beyond the dichotomy of short-term and long-term memory, researchers delve into the nuanced mechanisms underlying memory formation, retention, and retrieval.

Within the realm of long-term memory, researchers are increasingly focusing on the role of consolidation processes in shaping memory retention over time. Consolidation refers to the stabilization of memories, where initially fragile memories become more robust and resistant to forgetting.

Age-related changes in consolidation mechanisms, such as alterations in synaptic plasticity and neurotransmitter levels, may contribute to difficulties in forming enduring memories among older adults. Understanding these consolidation processes holds promise for developing interventions aimed at bolstering long-term memory in aging populations.

Moreover, recent studies have shed light on the impact of lifestyle factors on memory and cognitive aging. Engaging in mentally stimulating activities, such as puzzles, reading, or learning new skills, has been associated with better cognitive outcomes in older adults. The concept of cognitive reserve suggests that individuals who regularly challenge their brains may develop greater resilience to age-related cognitive decline. Encouraging lifelong learning and cognitive engagement may thus serve as a protective factor against memory decline in later life.

In addition to lifestyle factors, emerging research highlights the influence of social connectedness on cognitive aging and memory function. Maintaining strong social ties and engaging in social activities has been linked to better cognitive health and reduced risk of dementia. Social interaction provides cognitive stimulation, emotional support, and opportunities for intellectual engagement, all of which may contribute to preserved memory function in older age. Addressing social isolation and promoting community engagement may therefore represent important strategies for supporting cognitive vitality in aging populations.

Furthermore, advancements in neuroimaging techniques offer valuable insights into the neural underpinnings of age-related memory decline. Functional magnetic resonance imaging (fMRI), positron emission tomography (PET), and diffusion tensor imaging (DTI) allow researchers to examine structural and functional changes in the aging brain with unprecedented detail. These imaging modalities reveal alterations in brain connectivity, regional activity patterns, and neural network dynamics associated with age-related memory impairments. By elucidating the neurobiological basis of memory decline, neuroimaging studies contribute to the development of targeted interventions and personalized treatments for cognitive aging.

On a broader societal level, addressing ageism and promoting age-friendly environments are essential for supporting cognitive health and well-being in older adults. Ageism, or discrimination based on age, can perpetuate negative stereotypes and undermine the self-perception and confidence of older individuals. Combatting ageist attitudes and fostering inclusive communities that value the contributions of older adults can enhance social connectedness and promote active aging. Creating environments that facilitate access to healthcare, social services, and lifelong learning opportunities is crucial for promoting cognitive resilience and preserving memory function across the lifespan.

The relationship between memory and aging is multifaceted, encompassing a myriad of biological, psychological, and social factors. Understanding the complex interplay between these factors is essential for developing effective strategies to support cognitive health and well-being in older populations. By exploring the underlying mechanisms of memory decline, promoting lifestyle factors that foster cognitive resilience, harnessing the power of social connectedness, leveraging neuroimaging technologies, and challenging ageist attitudes, we can strive to create a society where aging is associated with vitality, wisdom, and continued cognitive engagement.

In the exploration of memory and aging, researchers are increasingly investigating the role of sleep in memory consolidation and cognitive function in older adults. Sleep plays a critical role in memory processing, with different stages of sleep implicated in various aspects of memory formation and retention. Age-related changes in sleep architecture, such as alterations in sleep duration, efficiency, and quality, may disrupt memory consolidation processes and contribute to cognitive decline. Understanding the interplay between sleep and memory in aging is essential for developing interventions aimed at optimizing sleep health and preserving cognitive function in older individuals.

Moreover, emerging evidence suggests that nutritional factors may influence memory and cognitive aging. Dietary patterns rich in antioxidants, omega-3 fatty acids, and other micronutrients have been associated with better cognitive performance and reduced risk of age-related cognitive decline. Conversely, diets high in saturated fats, refined sugars, and processed foods may have detrimental effects on brain health and memory function. Nutritional interventions, such as dietary supplementation and dietary counseling, hold promise for mitigating cognitive decline and promoting brain health in aging populations.

Another area of research focus is the potential role of neuroplasticity in mediating age-related changes in memory function. Neuroplasticity refers to the brain's ability to reorganize and adapt in response to environmental stimuli and experiences. While aging is often associated with declines in neuroplasticity, recent studies suggest that certain interventions, such as cognitive training, physical exercise, and environmental enrichment, may enhance neuroplasticity and promote cognitive resilience in older adults. By harnessing the brain's inherent plasticity, researchers aim to develop novel interventions to combat memory decline and promote healthy aging.

Furthermore, advances in genetics and molecular biology have uncovered genetic factors that may influence memory and cognitive aging. Genetic variants associated with neurodegenerative diseases, such as Alzheimer's disease, have been linked to alterations in memory function and brain structure in older adults. Understanding the genetic basis of memory decline may facilitate the development of personalized interventions and targeted treatments for individuals at risk of cognitive impairment. Genetic screening and counseling may also play a role in identifying individuals predisposed to memory disorders and guiding preventive strategies to optimize cognitive health.

In addition to genetic factors, epigenetic mechanisms have emerged as key regulators of memory function and cognitive aging. Epigenetic modifications, such as DNA methylation and histone acetylation, can modulate gene expression patterns in response to environmental stimuli and experiences. Age-related changes in epigenetic regulation may contribute to alterations in memory-related gene expression and neuronal function. Targeting epigenetic mechanisms holds promise for developing novel therapeutics to enhance memory function and mitigate cognitive decline in aging populations.

Moreover, recent advancements in artificial intelligence and machine learning have enabled researchers to analyze large-scale datasets and identify novel biomarkers of cognitive aging and memory impairment. By integrating multimodal data from neuroimaging, genetic, epigenetic, and other sources, researchers can develop predictive models to identify individuals at risk of cognitive decline and personalize interventions accordingly. Artificial intelligence algorithms may also facilitate the discovery of new therapeutic targets and treatment strategies for age-related memory disorders.

The study of memory and aging encompasses a diverse array of disciplines, including neuroscience, psychology, genetics, nutrition, and technology. By elucidating the complex mechanisms underlying memory decline and cognitive aging, researchers aim to develop holistic approaches to promote cognitive health and well-being in older populations. From lifestyle interventions to genetic and epigenetic therapies to artificial intelligence-driven innovations, the quest to understand and enhance memory function in aging is a multifaceted endeavor with profound implications for the future of aging societies.

Common memory problems associated with aging

Memory is a vital cognitive function that allows us to retain and recall information acquired through our experiences. However, as individuals age, they may experience various challenges and difficulties with memory, which can impact daily functioning and quality of life. Understanding the common memory problems associated with aging is essential for identifying potential interventions and strategies to support cognitive health in older adults.

One of the most prevalent memory problems in aging is forgetfulness, characterized by the inability to recall information or events accurately. Age-related forgetfulness may involve difficulties in remembering names, appointments, or where objects were placed. While occasional forgetfulness is considered normal, persistent and disruptive memory lapses may indicate underlying cognitive changes or conditions such as mild cognitive impairment (MCI) or dementia.

Another common memory problem associated with aging is prospective memory deficits, which involve difficulties in remembering to perform intended actions in the future. Older adults may struggle to remember appointments, take medication on time, or complete tasks at scheduled intervals. Prospective memory deficits can have significant implications for daily functioning and may result in missed appointments, medication errors, or difficulties in managing daily activities.

Memory, a cornerstone of cognitive function, serves as the repository of our life's experiences, enabling us to recall information crucial for navigating daily existence. Yet, as the years advance, individuals often encounter a myriad of challenges that assail this once steadfast faculty, impeding its efficacy and diminishing the quality of life. It is imperative to comprehend the spectrum of memory woes that accompany the aging process, as doing so holds the key to devising interventions and strategies that foster cognitive well-being among older demographics.

Forgetfulness stands as a towering sentinel among the myriad of memory tribulations that afflict the elderly populace. It manifests as a chronic inability to retrieve information or recollect events with precision, casting a shadow over one's ability to function seamlessly in everyday life. The aging mind grapples with a litany of forgetful episodes, from the trivial misplacement of objects to the disconcerting struggle to summon names and appointments from the recesses of memory. While sporadic memory lapses may be deemed innocuous, their incessant recurrence could portend deeper cognitive shifts or herald the onset of conditions such as mild cognitive impairment (MCI) or dementia.

Prospective memory, too, bears the brunt of the aging process, succumbing to a gradual erosion that impairs the individual's ability to execute planned actions in the future. This facet of memory governs our capacity to remember and fulfill intentions, whether it pertains to adhering to scheduled medication regimens, attending appointments, or completing tasks within stipulated timeframes. For older adults grappling with prospective memory deficits, the ramifications extend beyond mere inconvenience, permeating the fabric of daily life and culminating in missed engagements, medication mishaps, and a palpable struggle to orchestrate routine activities with precision.

Moreover, the aging mind contends with the insidious encroachment of episodic memory decline, a phenomenon marked by a faltering ability to recollect specific events and experiences from the past. Individuals find themselves ensnared in a labyrinth of fragmented recollections, wherein the threads of temporal continuity fray and unravel, leaving lacunae in the tapestry of personal history. The inexorable march of time exacts its toll on episodic memory, robbing older adults of the capacity to reminisce with clarity and relish the richness of their life's narrative.

Beyond the realm of individual tribulations, memory deficits in aging precipitate a cascade of societal ramifications that reverberate far and wide. The burden of caregiving falls disproportionately on family members and healthcare providers, who grapple with the exigencies of supporting individuals grappling with cognitive decline. As the prevalence of memory-related disorders burgeons with the aging demographic, healthcare systems strain under the weight of burgeoning caseloads, underscoring the urgent imperative for scalable interventions that alleviate the societal burden of memory decline.

In response to the burgeoning epidemic of memory deficits in aging, researchers and clinicians alike are spearheading concerted efforts to unravel the intricacies of cognitive decline and devise targeted interventions that arrest its inexorable advance. From pharmacological agents that bolster neurotransmitter function to cognitive training regimens that harness the brain's inherent plasticity, a panoply of therapeutic modalities holds promise in mitigating the ravages of memory decline and restoring cognitive vitality to aging minds.

Yet, amidst the fervent quest for pharmacological panaceas and cognitive elixirs, the significance of lifestyle factors in shaping cognitive health looms large. Engaging in regular physical exercise, adhering to a balanced diet rich in brain-boosting nutrients, and fostering social connections that stave off isolation wield transformative potential in fortifying cognitive resilience and mitigating the risk of memory decline in aging. Furthermore, the cultivation of intellectually stimulating pursuits, from lifelong learning endeavors to leisure activities that foster cognitive engagement, serves as a bulwark against the insidious encroachments of cognitive decline, empowering individuals to traverse the twilight years with grace and vitality.

In the crucible of aging, memory emerges as a fulcrum upon which the arc of individual autonomy and well-being hinges. While the specter of cognitive decline may cast a pall over the horizon, it is incumbent upon society to marshal its collective resources and forge a path towards cognitive vitality and resilience for all individuals traversing the temporal landscape of aging. Through a multifaceted approach that encompasses targeted interventions, lifestyle modifications, and societal support systems, we can aspire to usher in an era where aging is synonymous not with decline, but with the enduring cultivation of cognitive flourishing and fulfillment.

Within the intricate tapestry of aging, the narrative of memory unfolds in myriad shades, each hue reflecting the complex interplay of biological, psychological, and environmental factors that sculpt the contours of cognitive decline. Among the pantheon of memory maladies that besiege the aging mind, semantic memory impairment emerges as a formidable adversary, undermining the individual's capacity to retrieve factual knowledge and conceptual understanding. This erosion of semantic memory not only impairs academic and occupational pursuits but also impinges upon the individual's ability to navigate the nuances of everyday conversation and comprehend the intricacies of the world around them.

Furthermore, the specter of memory decline casts a shadow over the realms of emotional processing and regulation, ushering in a tempest of affective upheaval that disrupts the equilibrium of mental well-being. As the aging mind grapples with the vicissitudes of memory impairment, emotional resilience wanes, leaving individuals vulnerable to the ravages of depression, anxiety, and existential angst. The erosion of autobiographical memory, in particular, precipitates a profound sense of existential dislocation, as the threads of personal identity unravel, leaving individuals adrift in a sea of fragmented recollections and disjointed narratives.

In addition to the deleterious effects wrought upon individual cognition and emotional well-being, memory decline in aging exacts a profound toll on the fabric of interpersonal relationships and social cohesion. As cherished memories fade into oblivion and the contours of shared experiences blur, the bonds that bind families and communities together fray at the seams, yielding a landscape marked by loneliness, isolation, and estrangement. The erosion of memory serves as a potent catalyst for intergenerational dissonance, as the chasm between past and present widens, leaving younger generations bereft of the wisdom and ancestral knowledge that enrich the tapestry of human experience.

Moreover, memory deficits in aging engender profound disparities in access to healthcare and social support services, exacerbating existing inequities and perpetuating cycles of disadvantage among vulnerable populations. Marginalized communities, including racial and ethnic minorities, individuals with disabilities, and those residing in underserved regions, bear the brunt of memory-related disparities, confronting barriers to diagnosis, treatment, and supportive care that perpetuate cycles of cognitive decline and social exclusion. Addressing these entrenched disparities requires a multifaceted approach that encompasses targeted outreach initiatives, culturally competent healthcare delivery, and the equitable allocation of resources to underserved communities.

Amidst the labyrinthine corridors of memory decline, a beacon of hope emerges in the form of emerging technologies that hold promise in reshaping the landscape of cognitive healthcare and empowerment. From wearable devices that monitor cognitive function in real-time to digital therapeutics that deliver personalized interventions tailored to individual cognitive profiles, the arsenal of technological innovations offers a glimmer of hope in the fight against memory decline. Furthermore, virtual reality platforms and immersive storytelling experiences provide avenues for preserving and reimagining cherished memories, fostering intergenerational dialogue, and enriching the fabric of collective remembrance.

In the crucible of aging, memory emerges not merely as a repository of past experiences but as a crucible of identity, a testament to the richness and complexity of the human condition. As we navigate the labyrinthine pathways of memory decline, let us heed the clarion call to compassion and solidarity, forging a future where aging is synonymous not with decline but with the enduring cultivation of cognitive vitality, emotional resilience, and social connectedness. In the tapestry of memory, let us weave threads of empathy and understanding, embracing the diverse tapestry of human experience and affirming the inherent dignity and worth of every individual traversing the temporal landscape of aging.

In the mosaic of memory's decline, the intersectionality of factors such as socioeconomic status, educational attainment, and access to healthcare emerges as a defining feature, shaping the trajectory of cognitive decline and exacerbating existing disparities in outcomes. Individuals hailing from marginalized backgrounds are disproportionately burdened by the scourge of memory deficits, confronting barriers to early intervention, diagnostic ambiguity, and limited access to evidence-based treatments that perpetuate cycles of cognitive decline and social marginalization. Addressing these entrenched disparities necessitates a holistic approach that transcends the confines of traditional healthcare paradigms, embracing community-based interventions, advocacy efforts, and policy initiatives that dismantle structural barriers and foster inclusive environments conducive to cognitive well-being for all.

Furthermore, the burgeoning field of cognitive neuroscience offers tantalizing insights into the neural substrates of memory decline, unraveling the intricate tapestry of synaptic dysfunction, neuroinflammation, and amyloid deposition that underpin age-related cognitive impairment. From longitudinal neuroimaging studies that track the trajectory of brain aging to experimental interventions that modulate neural plasticity and promote neurogenesis, the frontiers of cognitive neuroscience hold promise in illuminating the pathophysiological mechanisms that govern memory decline and informing the development of targeted therapeutics that arrest its inexorable advance.

In parallel, the paradigm of person-centered care emerges as a guiding ethos in the provision of support and assistance to individuals grappling with memory deficits in aging. Rooted in principles of dignity, autonomy, and empowerment, person-centered care eschews a one-size-fits-all approach in favor of individualized interventions that honor the unique preferences, values, and lived experiences of each person. By fostering collaborative partnerships between healthcare providers, caregivers, and individuals themselves, person-centered care transcends the transactional nature of traditional care delivery, imbuing the caregiving journey with empathy, compassion, and mutual respect.

Moreover, the transformative power of interdisciplinary collaboration comes to the fore in the quest to combat memory decline and promote cognitive resilience in aging. By harnessing the collective expertise of neuroscientists, geriatricians, psychologists, social workers, and allied healthcare professionals, interdisciplinary teams can devise holistic care plans that address the multifaceted dimensions of memory impairment, integrating pharmacological, psychosocial, and lifestyle-based interventions into a cohesive framework of care. Through interdisciplinary collaboration, silos are dismantled, and innovative solutions emerge, heralding a paradigm shift in the provision of care for individuals navigating the complexities of memory decline in aging.

In the crucible of aging, memory emerges not merely as a harbinger of loss but as a vessel of resilience, a testament to the indomitable spirit of the human mind in its quest for meaning, connection, and transcendence. As we traverse the labyrinthine pathways of memory decline, let us embrace the inherent complexity and inherent dignity of every individual, fostering environments that nurture cognitive vitality, emotional well-being, and social connectedness across the lifespan. In the mosaic of memory's decline, let us weave threads of compassion, solidarity, and hope, affirming the intrinsic worth and enduring legacy of every person who embarks on the timeless journey of aging.

Chapter III. Neuroplasticity and Aging

Definition of neuroplasticity and its role in aging brains

Neuroplasticity, often referred to as brain plasticity, is a fundamental property of the brain that refers to its ability to adapt, reorganize, and change in response to internal and external stimuli. This dynamic process underlies learning, memory, and recovery from injury, and it plays a crucial role in shaping the structure and function of the brain throughout life. Understanding neuroplasticity and its implications for aging brains is essential for promoting cognitive health and well-being in older adults.

At its core, neuroplasticity involves changes in the strength and connectivity of neuronal connections, known as synapses, as well as structural alterations in neural circuits. These changes can occur at various levels of organization, from molecular and cellular mechanisms to larger-scale neural networks. Neuroplasticity is driven by a combination of factors, including neuronal activity, neurotransmitter release, gene expression, and environmental influences.

In the context of aging brains, neuroplasticity becomes particularly relevant as individuals experience changes in cognitive function and brain structure over time. While aging is often associated with declines in certain cognitive abilities, such as memory and processing speed, research has shown that the aging brain remains capable of remarkable plasticity and adaptation. Despite the presence of age-related changes, older adults retain the capacity to learn new skills, form new memories, and adapt to novel environments.

One of the key mechanisms underlying neuroplasticity in aging brains is synaptic plasticity, which refers to the ability of synapses to undergo changes in strength and efficacy in response to activity. Synaptic plasticity is mediated by processes such as long-term potentiation (LTP) and long-term depression (LTD), which involve alterations in the release of neurotransmitters and the responsiveness of postsynaptic receptors. These mechanisms play a critical role in learning and memory processes and can be modulated by factors such as experience, environmental enrichment, and pharmacological interventions.

Moreover, neuroplasticity in aging brains is not limited to synaptic changes but also encompasses structural remodeling and reorganization of neural circuits. Studies using neuroimaging techniques such as magnetic resonance imaging (MRI) have revealed that older adults can exhibit structural changes in brain regions involved in cognitive functions, such as the prefrontal cortex and hippocampus. These changes may reflect adaptive processes aimed at compensating for age-related declines in neuronal function or promoting efficient neural processing.

The role of neuroplasticity in aging brains extends beyond cognitive function to include sensory and motor systems as well. Research has shown that older adults can benefit from sensory and motor training interventions that promote plasticity in sensory areas of the brain, leading to improvements in perception, balance, and motor coordination. Similarly, interventions targeting cognitive functions such as memory and attention can induce neuroplastic changes in relevant brain regions, enhancing cognitive performance in older adults.

Neuroplasticity is a fundamental property of the brain that enables adaptation, learning, and recovery throughout life.

In aging brains, neuroplasticity remains a dynamic and malleable process, allowing older adults to continue learning and adapting to changing circumstances. By understanding the mechanisms underlying neuroplasticity and implementing strategies to promote adaptive brain changes, we can support cognitive health and well-being in older adults.

In the context of aging, neuroplasticity assumes heightened significance as individuals navigate cognitive function changes and structural transformations in the brain over time. Despite the common association of aging with declines in cognitive abilities like memory and processing speed, research underscores the enduring capacity of the aging brain for remarkable plasticity and adaptation. Despite age-related changes, older adults retain the ability to acquire new skills, forge fresh memories, and acclimate to novel environments.

Synaptic plasticity emerges as a pivotal mechanism underpinning neuroplasticity in aging brains. It denotes the synapses' capability to undergo alterations in strength and efficacy in response to activity. Processes like long-term potentiation (LTP) and long-term depression (LTD) mediate synaptic plasticity, involving shifts in neurotransmitter release and postsynaptic receptor responsiveness. These mechanisms are integral to learning and memory processes, modifiable by experiences, environmental enrichment, and pharmacological interventions.

In essence, neuroplasticity emerges as a foundational attribute of the brain, facilitating adaptation, learning, and recovery across the lifespan. In aging brains, neuroplasticity perseveres as a dynamic and adaptable process, empowering older adults to persist in learning and adjusting to evolving circumstances. By unraveling the mechanisms underpinning neuroplasticity and deploying strategies to foster adaptive brain changes, we can uphold cognitive health and overall well-being in the elderly population.

Moreover, recent advancements in neuroscience have shed light on the intricate mechanisms that orchestrate neuroplasticity in aging brains. For instance, studies have elucidated the role of neurotrophic factors, such as brain-derived neurotrophic factor (BDNF), in promoting synaptic plasticity and neuronal survival. BDNF, a protein crucial for the growth, development, and maintenance of neurons, has been found to decline with age. However, interventions like physical exercise have been shown to enhance BDNF levels, thereby facilitating neuroplasticity and cognitive function in older adults.

Additionally, emerging research suggests that lifestyle factors, including diet, sleep, and social engagement, exert profound influences on neuroplasticity and brain health in aging individuals. A diet rich in antioxidants, omega-3 fatty acids, and other nutrients has been linked to improved cognitive function and reduced risk of neurodegenerative diseases. Furthermore, adequate sleep plays a vital role in consolidating memories and facilitating synaptic plasticity, while social interaction and cognitive engagement stimulate neural networks, fostering resilience against age-related cognitive decline.

Furthermore, the exploration of non-invasive brain stimulation techniques, such as transcranial magnetic stimulation (TMS) and transcranial direct current stimulation (tDCS), has opened new avenues for enhancing neuroplasticity in aging brains. These techniques modulate neuronal activity in targeted brain regions, offering promising avenues for treating cognitive impairments associated with aging and neurodegenerative conditions.

While research in this field is still evolving, preliminary findings suggest the potential of brain stimulation as a tool for promoting cognitive resilience and well-being in older adults.

Moreover, the concept of "cognitive reserve" has garnered attention as a protective factor against cognitive decline in aging. Cognitive reserve refers to the brain's ability to withstand neuropathological damage through adaptive processes, such as neuroplasticity, or by utilizing alternative neural networks. Factors contributing to cognitive reserve include educational attainment, occupational complexity, and engagement in mentally stimulating activities. By bolstering cognitive reserve through lifelong learning and intellectual pursuits, individuals can potentially mitigate the impact of aging on cognitive function and maintain cognitive vitality in later life.

Furthermore, the integration of technology-based interventions holds promise for enhancing neuroplasticity and cognitive function in aging populations. Cognitive training programs, delivered through computerized tasks and interactive applications, have been shown to induce neuroplastic changes and improve cognitive abilities in older adults. Virtual reality platforms offer immersive environments for cognitive rehabilitation and sensory-motor training, promoting neural adaptation and functional recovery in aging brains.

Additionally, personalized approaches to promoting neuroplasticity in aging individuals are gaining traction within the field of precision medicine. By leveraging genetic, neuroimaging, and biomarker data, researchers aim to tailor interventions to individuals' specific neurobiological profiles, optimizing their efficacy and outcomes. This personalized approach holds the potential to revolutionize how we address cognitive aging, offering tailored solutions that harness the brain's inherent plasticity to maintain cognitive health and well-being in older adults.

Neuroplasticity stands as a dynamic and adaptive process that continues to shape the aging brain's structure and function. Understanding the mechanisms underlying neuroplasticity and harnessing its potential through lifestyle interventions, brain stimulation techniques, cognitive reserve-building activities, and personalized approaches can empower older adults to maintain cognitive vitality and quality of life as they age. By embracing neuroplasticity as a cornerstone of healthy aging, we can pave the way for a future where aging is characterized not by decline, but by resilience, growth, and lifelong learning.

Furthermore, interdisciplinary collaborations between neuroscientists, clinicians, psychologists, and gerontologists are essential for advancing our understanding of neuroplasticity in aging and translating research findings into practical interventions. By fostering partnerships across different fields, researchers can gain insights into the complex interplay between biological, psychological, and social factors influencing neuroplasticity and cognitive aging. This collaborative approach facilitates the development of holistic interventions that address the multifaceted nature of cognitive health in older adults.

Moreover, the exploration of novel therapeutic avenues, such as nutraceuticals and neuropharmacological agents, holds promise for enhancing neuroplasticity and cognitive function in aging populations. Nutraceuticals, including compounds like polyphenols, flavonoids, and omega-3 fatty acids, exhibit neuroprotective properties and may support synaptic plasticity and neuronal resilience. Similarly, pharmacological agents targeting neurotransmitter systems implicated in neuroplasticity, such as acetylcholine and glutamate, offer potential avenues for enhancing cognitive function and mitigating age-related cognitive decline.

Furthermore, adopting a lifespan approach to promoting neuroplasticity is crucial for optimizing cognitive health across the aging trajectory. Initiatives aimed at fostering neuroplasticity should begin in early and midlife stages, emphasizing the importance of maintaining brain health through healthy lifestyle practices, cognitive engagement, and social participation. By instilling habits conducive to neuroplasticity early on, individuals can build cognitive reserve and resilience that serve as protective factors against age-related cognitive decline later in life.

Additionally, addressing disparities in access to resources and healthcare services is imperative for promoting equitable opportunities for neuroplasticity and cognitive well-being among older adults. Socioeconomic factors, including income, education, and access to healthcare, profoundly influence individuals' ability to engage in activities that support neuroplasticity, such as lifelong learning, cognitive enrichment, and preventive healthcare. Efforts to reduce disparities and ensure equitable access to resources can enhance the cognitive resilience and quality of life of aging populations across diverse socioeconomic backgrounds.

Furthermore, fostering a culture that values and celebrates aging as a period of growth, wisdom, and continued learning is essential for promoting neuroplasticity and well-being among older adults. Combatting ageist stereotypes and promoting positive attitudes toward aging can empower older individuals to embrace opportunities for personal growth, skill development, and intellectual exploration. By fostering an age-friendly society that recognizes and supports the diverse capabilities and contributions of older adults, we can create environments conducive to promoting neuroplasticity and healthy cognitive aging.

Advancing our understanding of neuroplasticity and its implications for cognitive aging requires a multifaceted approach that integrates scientific research, clinical practice, public health initiatives, and societal attitudes toward aging. By harnessing the inherent plasticity of the aging brain through personalized interventions, interdisciplinary collaborations, and a lifespan perspective, we can empower older adults to maintain cognitive vitality and lead fulfilling lives as they age. Embracing neuroplasticity as a fundamental aspect of healthy aging holds the potential to transform our approach to aging from one focused on decline to one centered on resilience, growth, and lifelong learning.

Ways in which the aging brain can adapt and change

The aging brain is a remarkably adaptable organ, capable of undergoing changes in response to various internal and external factors. Despite the presence of age-related structural and functional changes, older adults retain the capacity for neuroplasticity, the brain's ability to reorganize and adapt throughout life. Understanding the ways in which the aging brain can adapt and change is essential for promoting cognitive health and well-being in older adults.

One of the primary ways in which the aging brain can adapt is through synaptic plasticity, the ability of synapses to strengthen or weaken in response to activity. Synaptic plasticity plays a crucial role in learning and memory processes and can be modulated by factors such as experience, environmental enrichment, and pharmacological interventions. Older adults can engage in activities that promote synaptic plasticity, such as learning new skills, engaging in social interactions, and participating in cognitive training programs.

Moreover, the aging brain can undergo structural changes and reorganization in response to cognitive stimulation and environmental enrichment. Research has shown that older adults who engage in mentally stimulating activities, such as reading, playing musical instruments, or learning a new language, exhibit increased gray matter volume and enhanced connectivity in brain regions associated with cognitive functions. These structural changes may reflect adaptive processes aimed at maintaining cognitive function and compensating for age-related declines.

In addition to cognitive stimulation, physical activity has been shown to promote neuroplasticity in the aging brain. Regular exercise has been associated with improvements in cognitive function, brain structure, and neural connectivity in older adults. Aerobic exercise, in particular, has been shown to enhance hippocampal volume, increase blood flow to the brain, and promote the release of neurotrophic factors that support neuronal growth and survival.

Furthermore, social engagement and emotional well-being play important roles in promoting neuroplasticity and cognitive health in older adults. Maintaining social connections, participating in meaningful activities, and fostering a positive outlook can have beneficial effects on brain function and cognitive performance. Studies have shown that older adults who report higher levels of social support and engagement exhibit better cognitive function and a reduced risk of cognitive decline.

Nutrition and lifestyle factors also influence neuroplasticity and brain health in aging. A balanced diet rich in antioxidants, omega-3 fatty acids, and other nutrients can support brain function and protect against age-related cognitive decline. Adequate sleep is essential for memory consolidation and cognitive performance, while stress management techniques such as mindfulness meditation can promote resilience and adaptive coping strategies.

The aging brain retains the capacity for adaptation and change, allowing older adults to maintain cognitive function and well-being despite age-related challenges. By engaging in activities that promote neuroplasticity, such as cognitive stimulation, physical exercise, social engagement, and healthy lifestyle choices, older adults can support brain health and preserve cognitive function as they age.

The human brain is an astonishingly adaptable organ, capable of undergoing transformations in response to various internal and external influences. As individuals age, the brain undergoes structural and functional alterations. However, it retains the remarkable capacity for neuroplasticity, which refers to the brain's ability to reorganize and adapt throughout life. Understanding the mechanisms by which the aging brain can adapt and change is crucial for promoting cognitive health and overall well-being in older adults.

Moreover, social engagement and emotional well-being play significant roles in fostering neuroplasticity and cognitive health in older adults. Sustaining social connections, participating in meaningful activities, and cultivating a positive outlook can positively impact brain function and cognitive performance. Studies have revealed that older adults who report higher levels of social support and engagement tend to exhibit better cognitive function and a reduced risk of cognitive decline.

Furthermore, emerging research suggests that certain interventions may hold promise in enhancing neuroplasticity and cognitive function in aging populations. For instance, cognitive training programs tailored to older adults have been developed to target specific cognitive abilities such as memory, attention, and executive functions. These programs often utilize computerized exercises and games designed to challenge and stimulate the brain. Studies investigating the efficacy of such interventions have shown promising results, with participants demonstrating improvements in cognitive performance and everyday functioning.

Additionally, non-invasive brain stimulation techniques, such as transcranial magnetic stimulation (TMS) and transcranial direct current stimulation (tDCS), have garnered attention for their potential to modulate neuroplasticity and enhance cognitive function in older adults. These techniques involve applying weak electrical currents or magnetic fields to specific regions of the brain, thereby influencing neuronal activity. While research in this area is still evolving, preliminary findings suggest that brain stimulation may offer a novel approach to augmenting neuroplasticity and cognitive resilience in aging populations.

Moreover, advances in neuroimaging technologies have provided unprecedented insights into the structural and functional changes occurring in the aging brain. Techniques such as magnetic resonance imaging (MRI), positron emission tomography (PET), and functional MRI (fMRI) allow researchers to visualize brain anatomy, activity, and connectivity with unprecedented detail. By studying these neuroimaging markers, scientists can better understand the mechanisms underlying neuroplasticity and identify potential targets for interventions aimed at preserving cognitive function in older adults.

Furthermore, genetic factors play a significant role in shaping individual differences in neuroplasticity and cognitive aging. Recent genome-wide association studies (GWAS) have identified genetic variants associated with cognitive performance and age-related cognitive decline. By elucidating the genetic underpinnings of neuroplasticity, researchers hope to uncover novel therapeutic targets and personalized interventions for maintaining cognitive health in aging populations.

In addition to individual interventions, public health initiatives aimed at promoting brain health and cognitive aging are gaining traction. Governments and healthcare organizations are increasingly recognizing the importance of addressing cognitive health as part of comprehensive aging strategies. Initiatives may include promoting lifelong learning opportunities, creating age-friendly environments that support social engagement and physical activity, and raising awareness about the importance of healthy lifestyle habits for maintaining cognitive function as individuals age.

Furthermore, interdisciplinary collaboration between neuroscientists, psychologists, geriatricians, and public health experts is essential for advancing our understanding of neuroplasticity and cognitive aging. By fostering collaboration and knowledge exchange across different disciplines, researchers can develop holistic approaches to promoting cognitive health and well-being in aging populations. This interdisciplinary approach may involve integrating insights from neuroscience, psychology, genetics, epidemiology, and public health to develop comprehensive interventions that address the multifaceted nature of cognitive aging.

While aging is associated with changes in brain structure and function, the aging brain retains a remarkable capacity for adaptation and change. By understanding the mechanisms underlying neuroplasticity and cognitive aging, researchers and healthcare professionals can develop targeted interventions to support brain health and preserve cognitive function in older adults. From cognitive training programs and brain stimulation techniques to public health initiatives and interdisciplinary collaboration, a multifaceted approach is essential for promoting cognitive resilience and well-being as individuals age.

Moreover, as the global population continues to age, addressing cognitive health and promoting successful aging has become a pressing public health priority. The World Health Organization (WHO) recognizes the importance of cognitive health in its Global Strategy and Action Plan on Aging and Health, which calls for comprehensive approaches to support older adults' cognitive well-being. Governments, policymakers, and healthcare systems worldwide are increasingly focused on implementing strategies to enhance cognitive resilience and quality of life in aging populations.

Innovative technologies also hold promise in supporting cognitive health and neuroplasticity in older adults. Virtual reality (VR) platforms, for example, have been explored as tools for cognitive rehabilitation and stimulation. VR environments can provide immersive experiences that challenge cognitive abilities, such as memory, attention, and spatial awareness, in a safe and engaging manner. Preliminary studies suggest that VR-based interventions may offer benefits for cognitive function and psychological well-being in older adults.

Furthermore, ongoing research is shedding light on the role of lifestyle factors in influencing neuroplasticity and cognitive aging trajectories. Factors such as socioeconomic status, education level, and occupational complexity have been linked to cognitive reserve, the brain's ability to withstand age-related changes and pathology. Individuals with higher cognitive reserve may exhibit better cognitive outcomes in later life, even in the presence of brain pathology. Understanding how lifestyle factors contribute to cognitive reserve can inform strategies to optimize brain health and resilience across the lifespan.

Additionally, interventions targeting modifiable risk factors for cognitive decline, such as cardiovascular health and metabolic function, hold promise in promoting cognitive resilience in aging populations. Lifestyle modifications, including dietary changes, regular physical activity, and management of cardiovascular risk factors (e.g., hypertension, diabetes), have been associated with improved cognitive outcomes and reduced risk of dementia. Comprehensive interventions that address both brain health and systemic health may offer synergistic benefits for cognitive aging.

Moreover, personalized approaches to cognitive health are gaining traction, driven by advances in precision medicine and digital health technologies. By leveraging genetic information, biomarkers, and digital health monitoring tools, healthcare providers can tailor interventions to individuals' unique risk profiles and cognitive needs. Personalized interventions may include targeted lifestyle recommendations, pharmacological interventions, and cognitive training programs tailored to optimize cognitive function and resilience in older adults.

Furthermore, the societal implications of cognitive aging extend beyond individual health outcomes, impacting families, communities, and healthcare systems. Age-friendly initiatives aim to create environments that support aging populations' cognitive health and independence, encompassing aspects such as accessible housing, transportation, and community services. By fostering age-friendly environments, societies can promote social inclusion, reduce disparities in cognitive health, and enhance the overall quality of life for older adults.

Addressing cognitive aging requires a multifaceted approach that encompasses individual interventions, public health initiatives, technological innovations, and societal efforts. By leveraging our growing understanding of neuroplasticity, cognitive reserve, and modifiable risk factors, we can develop comprehensive strategies to support brain health and cognitive resilience in aging populations. From personalized interventions to age-friendly environments, collaboration across sectors is essential for promoting cognitive well-being and ensuring that individuals can age successfully and maintain their cognitive abilities for as long as possible.

Strategies for promoting neuroplasticity in older adults

Promoting neuroplasticity in older adults is essential for maintaining cognitive function, preserving brain health, and enhancing overall well-being. Neuroplasticity, the brain's ability to reorganize and adapt throughout life, offers opportunities for older adults to continue learning, growing, and adapting to changing circumstances. Implementing strategies that support neuroplasticity can help older adults maintain cognitive vitality and independence as they age.

One effective strategy for promoting neuroplasticity in older adults is engaging in lifelong learning activities. Learning new skills, hobbies, or languages challenges the brain and stimulates neural networks involved in memory, attention, and problem-solving. Older adults can take advantage of community education programs, online courses, or local workshops to explore new interests and expand their cognitive horizons.

Physical exercise is another powerful tool for promoting neuroplasticity in aging brains. Aerobic exercise, in particular, has been shown to enhance brain function, improve cognitive performance, and promote the growth of new neurons in the hippocampus, a brain region critical for learning and memory. Older adults can incorporate regular exercise into their daily routine through activities such as walking, swimming, cycling, or group fitness classes.

Social engagement and meaningful relationships play a crucial role in promoting neuroplasticity and cognitive health in older adults. Maintaining social connections, participating in group activities, and volunteering can provide opportunities for intellectual stimulation, emotional support , and social interaction, all of which contribute to brain health and well-being. Joining clubs, attending community events, or participating in group activities can provide opportunities for social engagement and cognitive stimulation, fostering resilience and adaptive coping strategies in older adults.

Furthermore, cognitive training programs have been developed specifically to target cognitive functions and promote neuroplasticity in older adults. These programs often include exercises and activities designed to challenge memory, attention, and problem-solving skills. Computer-based cognitive training programs, in particular, have shown promise in improving cognitive function and promoting brain health in older adults.

In addition to cognitive stimulation and physical activity, maintaining a healthy lifestyle is essential for supporting neuroplasticity in aging brains. A balanced diet rich in fruits, vegetables, whole grains, and lean proteins provides essential nutrients that support brain function and protect against age-related cognitive decline. Adequate hydration is also important for brain health, as dehydration can impair cognitive performance and memory.

Moreover, managing stress and prioritizing relaxation can help older adults maintain cognitive vitality and support neuroplasticity. Stress management techniques such as mindfulness meditation, deep breathing exercises, and progressive muscle relaxation can reduce stress levels and promote emotional well-being. Prioritizing hobbies, leisure activities, and self-care can also contribute to overall brain health and resilience in older adults.

It's important for older adults to prioritize quality sleep, as sleep plays a crucial role in memory consolidation and cognitive function. Establishing a regular sleep schedule, creating a relaxing bedtime routine, and optimizing sleep environment can promote restful sleep and support brain health in aging. Avoiding caffeine and electronic devices before bedtime can also help improve sleep quality and cognitive function in older adults.

Promoting neuroplasticity in older adults is essential for maintaining cognitive vitality, preserving brain health, and enhancing overall well-being. By engaging in activities that stimulate the brain, such as lifelong learning, physical exercise, social engagement, and cognitive training, older adults can support neuroplasticity and adaptability in aging brains. Implementing healthy lifestyle habits, managing stress, prioritizing sleep, and practicing self-care further contribute to brain health and resilience in older adults. By incorporating these strategies into daily life, older adults can optimize cognitive function, maintain independence, and enjoy a fulfilling and vibrant later life.

Furthermore, ongoing efforts in research and development are exploring novel approaches to bolster cognitive health and neuroplasticity in aging individuals. One such avenue involves the investigation of dietary supplements and pharmacological agents that target mechanisms underlying neuroplasticity and cognitive function. Compounds such as flavonoids, found in foods like berries and dark chocolate, have shown promise in enhancing brain health and cognitive performance through their antioxidant and anti-inflammatory properties. Similarly, pharmaceutical agents targeting neurotransmitter systems implicated in learning and memory, such as acetylcholine and glutamate, are being studied for their potential to promote neuroplasticity and cognitive resilience in aging populations.

Moreover, holistic approaches to cognitive health encompass not only interventions targeting the brain but also those addressing psychosocial and environmental factors. Mental health support services, including counseling and therapy, play a crucial role in promoting emotional well-being and resilience in older adults. Addressing factors such as depression, anxiety, and stress can have profound effects on cognitive function and overall quality of life. Additionally, creating age-friendly communities that prioritize accessibility, social inclusion, and opportunities for engagement can enhance older adults' cognitive health and well-being.

Furthermore, the integration of technology into cognitive health interventions continues to evolve, with digital therapeutics and telehealth platforms offering new avenues for remote monitoring and intervention delivery. Mobile applications designed to promote cognitive fitness through brain training exercises, mindfulness practices, and cognitive assessments are increasingly accessible to older adults. Remote cognitive rehabilitation programs, delivered via telehealth platforms, provide opportunities for individuals to receive personalized support and guidance from healthcare professionals without the need for in-person visits.

Additionally, community-based programs and initiatives play a vital role in supporting cognitive health and social connectedness among older adults. Senior centers, adult education classes, and community centers offer opportunities for social interaction, lifelong learning, and engagement in meaningful activities. By fostering a sense of belonging and purpose, these programs contribute to cognitive stimulation and emotional well-being in aging populations. Collaborative efforts between healthcare providers, community organizations, and local governments are essential for developing and sustaining such initiatives.

Moreover, the promotion of brain-healthy lifestyles extends beyond individual behaviors to encompass broader environmental and policy changes. Urban planning strategies that prioritize walkable neighborhoods, green spaces, and access to recreational facilities can encourage physical activity and social engagement among older adults. Workplace policies that support lifelong learning, flexible retirement options, and age-friendly employment practices contribute to cognitive stimulation and financial security in later life.

The pursuit of cognitive health in aging populations requires a multifaceted and interdisciplinary approach that addresses biological, psychological, social, and environmental factors. Advances in research, technology, and public health policy offer promising opportunities to enhance neuroplasticity, cognitive resilience, and overall well-being in older adults. By fostering collaboration across sectors and leveraging innovative strategies, we can empower individuals to age successfully and maintain their cognitive vitality for as long as possible.

Furthermore, emerging research is exploring the potential role of environmental enrichment in promoting neuroplasticity and cognitive resilience in aging individuals. Environments that provide opportunities for novelty, complexity, and sensory stimulation have been shown to support brain health and cognitive function. Animal studies have demonstrated that enriched environments, characterized by increased social interaction, physical activity, and cognitive stimulation, can lead to structural and functional changes in the brain, including enhanced synaptic plasticity and neurogenesis. Translating these findings to human populations, interventions aimed at enriching living environments and promoting engagement in intellectually stimulating activities may offer benefits for cognitive aging.

Additionally, interventions targeting sleep quality and sleep-related disorders are gaining attention as potential avenues for preserving cognitive function in older adults. Poor sleep quality, characterized by disturbances in sleep duration, continuity, and architecture, has been associated with cognitive decline and an increased risk of neurodegenerative diseases. Interventions such as cognitive behavioral therapy for insomnia (CBT-I) and mindfulness-based approaches to sleep improvement have shown promise in improving sleep quality and cognitive outcomes in older adults. By addressing sleep disturbances and promoting healthy sleep habits, healthcare providers can support cognitive health and overall well-being in aging populations.

Moreover, the role of cultural factors and social determinants of health in shaping cognitive aging trajectories cannot be overlooked. Cultural attitudes toward aging, societal expectations, and access to resources influence individuals' opportunities for cognitive stimulation, social engagement, and healthcare access. Recognizing and addressing disparities in cognitive health outcomes among diverse populations is essential for promoting health equity and ensuring that all individuals have the opportunity to age with dignity and cognitive vitality.

Furthermore, the intersection between cognitive health and chronic disease management is an area of growing importance in geriatric care. Older adults living with chronic conditions such as diabetes, cardiovascular disease, and chronic pain often face additional challenges related to cognitive impairment and dementia risk. Integrated care models that address both physical and cognitive health needs, such as collaborative care teams and multidisciplinary clinics, are emerging as promising approaches to managing complex health issues in aging populations. By providing comprehensive, person-centered care, healthcare systems can optimize outcomes and enhance quality of life for older adults living with chronic conditions.

Additionally, ongoing efforts to enhance public awareness and understanding of cognitive aging are essential for promoting early intervention and prevention strategies.

Educational campaigns, community outreach initiatives, and public health messaging can help dispel myths and misconceptions about cognitive aging and dementia, reduce stigma, and empower individuals to take proactive steps to maintain brain health. By promoting brain-healthy behaviors and fostering a culture of lifelong learning and cognitive engagement, societies can support individuals in optimizing their cognitive function and well-being across the lifespan.

The pursuit of cognitive health in aging populations requires a comprehensive and interdisciplinary approach that addresses the complex interplay of biological, psychological, social, and environmental factors. From environmental enrichment and sleep interventions to cultural competency and chronic disease management, a diverse array of strategies is needed to support cognitive resilience and promote healthy aging. By prioritizing research, policy, and public awareness efforts, we can advance our understanding of cognitive aging and develop effective interventions to enhance quality of life for older adults around the world.

Moreover, emerging research is delving into the potential role of brain-computer interfaces (BCIs) in enhancing cognitive function and promoting neuroplasticity in aging populations. BCIs enable direct communication between the brain and external devices, offering opportunities for cognitive training, rehabilitation, and augmentation. By leveraging neurofeedback techniques, individuals can learn to modulate their brain activity patterns, fostering neuroplastic changes associated with improved cognitive performance. While still in early stages of development, BCIs hold promise as innovative tools for enhancing cognitive resilience and supporting healthy aging.

Furthermore, psychosocial interventions that target loneliness and social isolation have garnered attention for their potential impact on cognitive health in older adults. Loneliness has been linked to cognitive decline, dementia risk, and poor mental health outcomes, highlighting the importance of addressing social connectedness as a component of cognitive aging interventions. Interventions such as group-based activities, peer support programs, and community engagement initiatives aim to combat social isolation and promote meaningful social connections, thereby supporting cognitive health and well-being in aging populations.

Additionally, the integration of arts-based interventions into cognitive health promotion efforts represents a creative approach to stimulating neuroplasticity and enhancing cognitive function in older adults. Activities such as music therapy, visual arts programs, and dance/movement interventions offer opportunities for cognitive engagement, emotional expression, and social interaction. Research suggests that participation in arts-based activities can lead to improvements in cognitive performance, mood, and quality of life in older adults, underscoring the potential of the arts as a therapeutic modality for supporting cognitive aging.

Moreover, efforts to promote lifelong learning and cognitive engagement extend beyond formal educational settings to include informal learning opportunities and community-based programs. Lifelong learning initiatives, such as continuing education classes, adult learning centers, and online courses, provide avenues for older adults to pursue intellectual interests, acquire new skills, and engage in cognitive stimulation. By fostering a culture of curiosity and intellectual curiosity, lifelong learning initiatives contribute to cognitive reserve and support cognitive health throughout the aging process.

Furthermore, interventions targeting mental health and emotional well-being play a crucial role in promoting cognitive resilience in older adults. Psychosocial interventions such as cognitive-behavioral therapy (CBT), mindfulness-based stress reduction (MBSR), and positive psychology interventions aim to enhance coping skills, reduce stress, and cultivate emotional resilience in the face of age-related challenges. By addressing psychological factors that contribute to cognitive decline, these interventions empower older adults to maintain cognitive function and adaptively manage age-related changes.

Additionally, efforts to integrate cognitive health promotion into primary care settings are essential for reaching older adults and addressing cognitive health needs in a holistic manner. Screening tools, assessments, and preventive interventions embedded within primary care practices enable healthcare providers to identify cognitive concerns early, offer personalized interventions, and monitor cognitive health over time. By integrating cognitive health into routine healthcare encounters, primary care providers can play a pivotal role in promoting cognitive resilience and supporting healthy aging in their older adult patients.

The pursuit of cognitive health in aging populations necessitates a multifaceted and innovative approach that encompasses technological advances, psychosocial interventions, arts-based programs, lifelong learning initiatives, mental health support, and primary care integration. By leveraging diverse strategies and collaborating across disciplines, stakeholders can advance our understanding of cognitive aging and develop effective interventions to enhance cognitive resilience and quality of life for older adults. From brain-computer interfaces to community-based arts programs, a continuum of interventions is needed to support cognitive health and well-being across the lifespan.

Chapter IV. Brain Health and Lifestyle Factors

Importance of lifestyle factors in brain health and aging

In the pursuit of healthy aging, lifestyle factors play a pivotal role, particularly concerning brain health. As individuals age, the brain undergoes various changes, including structural and functional alterations. Lifestyle choices significantly influence these changes, with certain habits promoting cognitive vitality while others may accelerate cognitive decline.

Research suggests that maintaining an active and intellectually stimulating lifestyle can help preserve cognitive function as people age. Engaging in activities such as reading, puzzles, and learning new skills can promote neuroplasticity, the brain's ability to adapt and reorganize itself. This adaptive capacity is crucial for offsetting age-related cognitive decline.

Furthermore, regular physical exercise has been shown to have profound benefits for brain health. Exercise increases blood flow to the brain, delivering essential nutrients and oxygen while promoting the release of neurotransmitters that support mood and cognitive function. Moreover, physical activity stimulates the production of brain-derived neurotrophic factor (BDNF), a protein that enhances the growth and survival of neurons.

A balanced diet is another critical component of brain health. Certain nutrients, such as omega-3 fatty acids found in fish, antioxidants present in fruits and vegetables, and vitamins like B12 and folate, are particularly beneficial for cognitive function. Conversely, diets high in processed foods, saturated fats, and sugar may contribute to inflammation and oxidative stress, damaging brain cells and impairing cognitive performance.

Quality sleep is essential for brain health and overall well-being. During sleep, the brain consolidates memories, clears toxins, and facilitates neural repair processes. Chronic sleep deprivation has been linked to cognitive deficits, mood disturbances, and an increased risk of neurodegenerative diseases such as Alzheimer's. Establishing a consistent sleep schedule and creating a conducive sleep environment are key strategies for promoting optimal brain function.

Moreover, managing stress is crucial for maintaining brain health as we age. Prolonged stress can lead to the dysregulation of stress hormones, such as cortisol, which may impair memory, attention, and decision-making abilities. Adopting stress-reduction techniques such as mindfulness meditation, deep breathing exercises, and regular relaxation practices can help mitigate the negative impact of stress on the brain.

Lifestyle factors exert a profound influence on brain health and aging. By prioritizing activities that promote cognitive stimulation, engaging in regular exercise, consuming a nutritious diet, prioritizing quality sleep, and effectively managing stress, individuals can support brain function throughout the aging process. Embracing a holistic approach to wellness empowers individuals to optimize their cognitive vitality and enjoy a fulfilling and meaningful life as they grow older.

Lifestyle factors wield considerable influence over brain health and the aging process. By prioritizing activities that stimulate cognition, engaging in regular physical activity, adopting a nutrient-rich diet, ensuring adequate sleep, and implementing stress-management strategies, individuals can safeguard their cognitive faculties as they journey through life. Embracing a holistic approach to wellness empowers individuals to cultivate cognitive vitality and embrace the later stages of life with fulfillment and purpose.

Moreover, social interaction emerges as another crucial aspect of promoting brain health and resilience against aging. Maintaining strong social connections and engaging in meaningful relationships have been linked to better cognitive function and a reduced risk of cognitive decline. Regular social engagement provides mental stimulation, emotional support, and opportunities for learning and growth, all of which contribute to overall brain health.

In addition to mental and physical activities, lifelong learning plays a pivotal role in supporting cognitive vitality as individuals age. Continuously challenging the brain with new information and experiences helps to create and strengthen neural connections, fostering cognitive flexibility and resilience. Whether through formal education, online courses, or simply pursuing new hobbies and interests, the pursuit of knowledge can have profound benefits for brain health.

Furthermore, incorporating mindfulness practices into daily life can significantly enhance brain function and overall well-being. Mindfulness involves paying deliberate attention to the present moment without judgment, which has been shown to reduce stress, improve mood, and enhance cognitive abilities such as attention and memory. Regular mindfulness practice can lead to structural changes in the brain associated with improved emotional regulation and cognitive performance.

Another crucial factor in maintaining brain health is the avoidance of harmful substances, such as excessive alcohol consumption and illicit drug use. Alcohol abuse can have detrimental effects on brain structure and function, impairing cognitive abilities and increasing the risk of conditions such as dementia. Similarly, the use of illicit drugs can lead to neurochemical imbalances and structural damage in the brain, resulting in cognitive deficits and other neurological problems.

Moreover, engaging in activities that promote brain health is not only beneficial for individuals but also for society as a whole. As populations around the world continue to age, the prevalence of age-related cognitive decline and neurodegenerative diseases is expected to rise. By promoting healthy lifestyle choices and providing access to resources that support brain health, communities can reduce the burden of cognitive impairment and improve the quality of life for older adults.

Maintaining brain health is a multifaceted endeavor that requires a holistic approach encompassing various lifestyle factors. From mental stimulation and physical exercise to nutrition, sleep, stress management, social engagement, and mindfulness, each aspect plays a crucial role in supporting cognitive function and resilience against aging. By prioritizing these factors and making informed choices, individuals can optimize their brain health and enjoy a fulfilling and meaningful life as they age. Additionally, efforts to promote brain health at the community level can have far-reaching benefits, contributing to healthier and more vibrant societies in the face of an aging population.

Furthermore, emerging research suggests that environmental factors, such as exposure to nature and green spaces, can also influence brain health and cognitive function. Spending time in natural environments has been associated with reduced stress levels, improved mood, and enhanced cognitive performance. Nature walks, gardening, and outdoor activities offer opportunities for relaxation and mental rejuvenation, contributing to overall well-being and brain resilience.

Moreover, the integration of technology into daily life presents both opportunities and challenges for brain health in the digital age. While technology can provide access to valuable information and cognitive training tools, excessive screen time and digital overload may have adverse effects on brain function. Excessive use of smartphones, computers, and other digital devices has been linked to attention difficulties, reduced cognitive flexibility, and changes in brain structure, particularly in younger individuals. Therefore, striking a balance between technology use and offline activities is essential for maintaining optimal brain health in today's interconnected world.

Additionally, engaging in creative pursuits can foster cognitive stimulation and promote brain health throughout the lifespan. Activities such as painting, drawing, writing, music, and dance stimulate different areas of the brain, encouraging neural plasticity and creativity. Creative expression allows individuals to tap into their imagination, problem-solving skills, and emotional processing abilities, all of which contribute to cognitive vitality and well-being.

Furthermore, the role of genetics in brain health and aging cannot be overlooked. While lifestyle factors play a significant role in shaping cognitive outcomes, genetic predispositions also influence an individual's susceptibility to age-related cognitive decline and neurodegenerative diseases. Understanding one's genetic risk factors can inform personalized strategies for brain health, such as targeted interventions and early detection of potential cognitive impairments.

Moreover, access to quality healthcare and support services is essential for promoting brain health and addressing age-related cognitive challenges. Regular medical check-ups, cognitive assessments, and access to specialist care can help identify and manage risk factors for cognitive decline, ensuring timely intervention and support. Additionally, community-based programs and resources for older adults, such as senior centers, memory clinics, and support groups, provide valuable social connections and resources for maintaining cognitive function and overall well-being.

Promoting brain health and resilience against aging requires a comprehensive approach that addresses various lifestyle factors, environmental influences, genetic predispositions, and access to healthcare and support services. By embracing a holistic perspective and adopting strategies that encompass mental, physical, social, and environmental well-being, individuals can optimize their cognitive function and quality of life as they age. Moreover, ongoing research and community efforts are essential for advancing our understanding of brain health and developing innovative approaches to support healthy aging and cognitive vitality for all.

Furthermore, the importance of maintaining cognitive reserves throughout life cannot be overstated. Cognitive reserve refers to the brain's ability to withstand age-related changes and pathology through various compensatory mechanisms. Factors such as higher education, occupational complexity, and engagement in mentally stimulating activities contribute to the development of cognitive reserve, which can buffer against cognitive decline and delay the onset of dementia in later life. Therefore, lifelong learning and intellectual enrichment are essential for building and preserving cognitive reserves, ensuring resilience against age-related cognitive changes.

Additionally, promoting brain health requires addressing disparities in access to resources and opportunities that can influence cognitive outcomes. Socioeconomic factors, such as income, education, and access to healthcare, significantly impact brain health disparities among older adults. Individuals from disadvantaged backgrounds may face barriers to accessing quality education, nutritious food, healthcare services, and safe living environments, which can exacerbate the risk of cognitive decline and neurodegenerative diseases. Addressing these disparities through policies and programs that promote equitable access to education, healthcare, and social services is crucial for improving brain health outcomes and reducing health inequities in aging populations.

Furthermore, fostering a supportive and age-friendly environment is essential for promoting brain health and well-being in older adults. Age-friendly communities are designed to support the needs and preferences of older residents, enabling them to age in place with dignity and independence. Features such as accessible housing, transportation options, outdoor spaces, community centers, and social activities cater to the diverse needs of older adults, facilitating social engagement, physical activity, and cognitive stimulation. By creating environments that promote social inclusion, physical activity, and lifelong learning, communities can enhance the cognitive resilience and quality of life of their aging populations.

Moreover, the role of lifelong relationships and social networks in promoting brain health cannot be overstated. Maintaining close relationships with family, friends, and community members provides emotional support, reduces social isolation, and promotes mental well-being, all of which are essential for brain health. Regular social interactions stimulate cognitive function, enhance mood, and contribute to overall resilience against age-related cognitive decline. Therefore, fostering strong social connections and supportive relationships is vital for promoting brain health and successful aging.

Promoting brain health and cognitive resilience in aging populations requires a multifaceted approach that addresses individual lifestyle factors, environmental influences, genetic predispositions, access to resources, and social determinants of health. By prioritizing lifelong learning, intellectual enrichment, access to healthcare, social inclusion, and age-friendly environments, societies can support older adults in maintaining cognitive vitality and quality of life as they age. Moreover, advancing research, policies, and community initiatives aimed at promoting brain health and addressing health disparities is essential for ensuring that all individuals have the opportunity to age with dignity, independence, and optimal brain function.

Impact of diet, exercise, sleep, and stress on brain function

The interplay between diet, exercise, sleep, and stress profoundly impacts brain function, influencing cognitive performance, mood regulation, and overall mental well-being. Each of these lifestyle factors plays a distinct yet interconnected role in shaping brain health, highlighting the importance of adopting a holistic approach to wellness.

Diet serves as the foundation for brain function, providing essential nutrients that support neural growth, repair, and communication. Omega-3 fatty acids, found abundantly in fatty fish such as salmon and walnuts, are critical for maintaining the structural integrity of brain cell membranes and promoting synaptic plasticity. Antioxidants, found in colorful fruits and vegetables, combat oxidative stress and inflammation, safeguarding brain cells from damage.

Regular physical exercise is not only beneficial for cardiovascular health but also exerts profound effects on brain function. Aerobic exercise increases blood flow to the brain, delivering oxygen and nutrients essential for optimal cognitive function. Moreover, exercise stimulates the release of neurotransmitters such as dopamine and serotonin, which enhance mood and cognitive performance. Additionally, exercise promotes the production of brain-derived neurotrophic factor (BDNF), a protein that supports the growth and survival of neurons, fostering neuroplasticity and resilience.

Quality sleep is essential for cognitive consolidation and emotional regulation. During sleep, the brain consolidates memories, clears metabolic waste products, and facilitates neural repair processes. Adequate sleep duration and quality are crucial for maintaining attention, memory, and problem-solving abilities. Chronic sleep deprivation disrupts these essential functions, impairing cognitive performance and increasing the risk of mood disorders and neurodegenerative diseases.

Furthermore, chronic stress poses a significant threat to brain function, precipitating structural and functional changes in key brain regions involved in emotion regulation and cognitive control. Prolonged exposure to stress hormones such as cortisol can damage brain cells, impair synaptic connections, and compromise neuroplasticity. Stress management techniques such as mindfulness meditation, deep breathing exercises, and progressive muscle relaxation can mitigate the negative impact of stress on the brain, promoting emotional resilience and cognitive flexibility.

The integration of diet, exercise, sleep, and stress management is essential for optimizing brain function and promoting overall well-being. By prioritizing a balanced diet rich in nutrients, engaging in regular physical activity, prioritizing restorative sleep, and adopting effective stress management strategies, individuals can support cognitive vitality and emotional resilience throughout life. Embracing a lifestyle that nourishes the mind and body empowers individuals to thrive mentally, emotionally, and physically.
The intricate dance among diet, exercise, sleep, and stress wields significant influence over brain function, dictating cognitive prowess, emotional equilibrium, and the broader landscape of mental wellness. These components, though distinct in their mechanisms, intertwine seamlessly to sculpt the terrain of brain health, underscoring the imperative of embracing a comprehensive approach to holistic well-being.

In synthesis, the fusion of dietary prudence, physical exertion, restorative slumber, and judicious stress management emerges as an indispensable panacea for nurturing cerebral vitality and fostering holistic well-being. Through the cultivation of a dietary tapestry rich in nourishing constituents, the embrace of an active lifestyle, the prioritization of rejuvenating sleep, and the cultivation of stress-alleviating practices, individuals inscribe a narrative of cognitive robustness and emotional flourishing across the arc of their lives. In sowing the seeds of a lifestyle that nurtures both mind and body, individuals embark on a journey towards mental buoyancy, emotional equilibrium, and physical vibrancy.

Within the intricate tapestry of human existence, the symbiotic interplay between diet, exercise, sleep, and stress management emerges as the fulcrum upon which cognitive vitality and emotional resilience pivot. Each facet, while distinct in its modus operandi, converges harmoniously to shape the contours of brain health, underscoring the indispensability of a multifaceted approach to holistic well-being.

Diet, often regarded as the cornerstone of physical wellness, assumes an equally pivotal role in nurturing cognitive prowess and emotional equilibrium. The mosaic of nutrients gleaned from a diverse array of foods furnishes the brain with the raw materials requisite for sustained neuronal vigor and synaptic plasticity. Notably, micronutrients such as vitamins B6, B12, and folate wield profound influence over cognitive function, participating in neurotransmitter synthesis and homocysteine metabolism. Moreover, emerging evidence underscores the pivotal role of gut microbiota in modulating brain health, highlighting the importance of dietary diversity in fostering a flourishing microbial ecosystem within the gut-brain axis.

In tandem with dietary considerations, the rhythm of physical exertion orchestrates a symphony of physiological adaptations that reverberate deeply within the recesses of the brain. The cadence of aerobic exercise, in particular, emerges as a potent elixir for cerebral vitality, amplifying cerebral blood flow and engendering a milieu conducive to neurogenesis and synaptic pruning. Notably, recent studies elucidate the cognitive benefits accruing from resistance training, which not only fortifies musculoskeletal integrity but also galvanizes cognitive function through mechanisms involving neurotrophic factors and insulin-like growth factor 1 (IGF-1).

Amidst the ebb and flow of daily life, the sanctuary of sleep stands as a non-negotiable sanctuary for cognitive consolidation and emotional convalescence. The cyclical oscillations of REM (rapid eye movement) and non-REM sleep stages orchestrate a delicate choreography of neural processes, facilitating memory consolidation, emotional regulation, and the clearance of metabolic byproducts. Disturbances in sleep architecture, whether precipitated by intrinsic factors like sleep disorders or extrinsic stressors, exact a toll on cognitive acuity and emotional resilience, underscoring the imperative of prioritizing sleep hygiene as a cornerstone of brain health.

Concomitant with the rhythms of wakefulness and slumber, the specter of chronic stress casts a pervasive shadow over cerebral well-being, precipitating a cascade of maladaptive neurobiological alterations. The protracted surge of stress hormones, typified by the release of cortisol from the adrenal glands, engenders structural and functional aberrations within the amygdala, hippocampus, and prefrontal cortex— key bastions governing emotional regulation and cognitive control. In the crucible of chronic stress, the delicate equilibrium between excitatory and inhibitory neurotransmission falters, culminating in a dysregulated neuronal milieu characterized by heightened vulnerability to mood disorders and cognitive decline.

In navigating the labyrinthine terrain of modern existence, the cultivation of stress-alleviating practices assumes paramount importance as a bulwark against the deleterious incursions of chronic stress. Mindfulness meditation, with its emphasis on present-moment awareness and non-judgmental acceptance, emerges as a potent antidote to the tumult of ruminative thought patterns and emotional turbulence. Likewise, the rhythmic cadence of deep breathing exercises and the somatic grounding of progressive muscle relaxation serve as conduits for attenuating physiological arousal and fostering emotional equanimity amidst the tempest of daily stressors.

In summation, the harmonious integration of dietary mindfulness, physical exertion, restorative sleep, and judicious stress management embodies a paradigm of holistic well-being conducive to fostering cognitive vitality and emotional resilience. Through the cultivation of lifestyle practices that nurture both mind and body, individuals inscribe a narrative of flourishing across the arc of their lives, transcending the confines of mere existence to embrace a holistic ethos of thriving. In the pursuit of cognitive robustness and emotional equilibrium, the journey unfolds not as a destination, but as an ongoing odyssey guided by the beacon of self-care and mindful living.

Furthermore, the impact of lifestyle factors on brain health extends beyond individual well-being to encompass broader societal implications. In an era characterized by burgeoning rates of cognitive decline and mental health disorders, the imperative of adopting proactive measures to safeguard brain health assumes heightened urgency. Indeed, the burgeoning prevalence of neurodegenerative maladies like Alzheimer's disease underscores the imperative of prioritizing brain health as a public health priority.

Within the educational landscape, the recognition of lifestyle interventions as potent modulators of cognitive function heralds a paradigm shift in pedagogical approaches. Integrating physical activity breaks, mindfulness practices, and nutritious meal options within educational curricula not only augments academic performance but also fosters a conducive environment for holistic development. Likewise, within corporate settings, initiatives aimed at promoting employee well-being through wellness programs and stress management seminars yield tangible dividends in terms of productivity, job satisfaction, and employee retention.

Furthermore, as we delve deeper into the intricate nexus between lifestyle factors and brain health, it becomes evident that the ramifications extend far beyond individual well-being, permeating societal structures and cultural norms. In an era characterized by the relentless march of technological advancement and the frenetic pace of modern living, the imperative of prioritizing brain health assumes heightened urgency as a linchpin of societal resilience and collective flourishing.

Likewise, within corporate settings, initiatives aimed at promoting employee well-being through comprehensive wellness programs and stress management seminars yield tangible dividends in terms of productivity, job satisfaction, and organizational cohesion. By fostering a culture of well-being that prioritizes the holistic welfare of employees, organizations cultivate a workforce imbued with a sense of purpose, resilience, and intrinsic motivation—a potent recipe for sustained success in an increasingly competitive landscape.

Moreover, within healthcare systems, the integration of lifestyle medicine principles alongside traditional pharmacological interventions represents a paradigmatic shift in the delivery of healthcare services. By acknowledging the pivotal role of lifestyle factors in shaping health outcomes, healthcare providers can move beyond a narrow disease-centric approach to embrace a more holistic model of care—one that empowers individuals to reclaim agency over their health through informed decision-making and proactive self-care practices.

Indeed, the burgeoning prevalence of chronic diseases—ranging from cardiovascular disorders to metabolic syndromes—underscores the imperative of adopting a proactive stance towards health promotion and disease prevention. By leveraging the transformative potential of lifestyle interventions, healthcare systems can attenuate the burgeoning burden of chronic diseases, thereby alleviating strain on healthcare resources and enhancing overall population health outcomes.

In essence, the integration of dietary mindfulness, physical exertion, restorative sleep, and stress management practices embodies a holistic ethos of well-being that transcends the confines of individual experience to encompass broader societal implications. By recognizing the interconnectedness of human health with environmental, social, and economic factors, societies can forge a path towards a future characterized by resilience, vitality, and flourishing for all.

The intricate nexus between lifestyle factors and brain health underscores the imperative of adopting a holistic approach to well-being—one that acknowledges the interplay between individual choices, societal structures, and cultural norms. By harnessing the synergistic potential of lifestyle interventions, individuals and societies alike can cultivate a reservoir of cognitive vitality and emotional resilience capable of withstanding the myriad challenges of the modern world. In embracing a paradigm of proactive self-care and collective empowerment, we embark on a journey towards a future where brain health serves as the cornerstone of societal flourishing and human potential reaches unprecedented heights. Integration of lifestyle medicine principles alongside pharmacological interventions represents a paradigmatic departure from the conventional disease-centric model of care. By empowering individuals with the knowledge and tools requisite for self-care, healthcare providers can catalyze transformative changes in health behaviors, thereby mitigating the burgeoning burden of chronic diseases and enhancing overall quality of life.

The intricate nexus between lifestyle factors and brain health underscores the imperative of embracing a holistic approach to well-being. By harnessing the synergistic potential of dietary mindfulness, physical exertion, restorative sleep, and stress management practices, individuals can fortify cognitive vitality and foster emotional resilience across the lifespan. Moreover, the recognition of lifestyle interventions as potent modulators of brain health holds profound implications for education, corporate wellness initiatives, and healthcare delivery systems, underscoring the transformative power of proactive measures in safeguarding brain health and promoting flourishing societies.

Tips for maintaining a healthy brain as we age

As individuals age, preserving brain health becomes increasingly important for maintaining cognitive vitality and quality of life. Fortunately, there are several strategies that can help promote a healthy brain and mitigate age-related cognitive decline. By incorporating these tips into daily life, individuals can optimize brain function and enjoy a fulfilling and meaningful aging process.

1. Stay mentally active: Engage in activities that challenge the mind, such as puzzles, crosswords, reading, and learning new skills. Intellectual stimulation promotes neuroplasticity,

the brain's ability to adapt and reorganize itself, which is essential for maintaining cognitive function as we age.

2. Maintain a balanced diet: Consume a diet rich in fruits, vegetables, whole grains, lean proteins, and healthy fats. Include foods that are high in omega-3 fatty acids, antioxidants, vitamins, and minerals, which support brain health and protect against age-related cognitive decline.

3. Prioritize physical exercise: Incorporate regular aerobic exercise, strength training, and flexibility exercises into your routine. Physical activity increases blood flow to the brain, promotes the release of neurotransmitters that enhance mood and cognition, and stimulates the production of brain-derived neurotrophic factor (BDNF), a protein that supports neuronal growth and survival.

4. Get quality sleep: Aim for seven to nine hours of sleep per night and establish a consistent sleep schedule. Create a relaxing bedtime routine and optimize your sleep environment to promote restorative sleep. Quality sleep is essential for memory consolidation, emotional regulation, and overall brain health.

5. Manage stress effectively: Practice stress-reduction techniques such as mindfulness meditation, deep breathing exercises, and progressive muscle relaxation. Prioritize self-care activities that promote relaxation and emotional well-being. Chronic stress can impair cognitive function and increase the risk of age-related neurodegenerative diseases, so it's important to find healthy ways to cope with stress.

6. Stay socially connected: Maintain strong social connections with friends, family, and community members. Engage in meaningful social activities and cultivate supportive relationships. Social interaction promotes

cognitive stimulation, emotional resilience, and overall well-being, which are essential for healthy aging.

7. Challenge your brain: Continuously seek out new experiences and learning opportunities. Take up hobbies, pursue interests, and explore unfamiliar subjects. Challenging your brain with novel activities stimulates neural pathways and enhances cognitive reserve, which can help protect against cognitive decline in later life.

As we journey through life, the importance of maintaining brain health becomes increasingly evident, particularly as we age. Preserving cognitive vitality is not just about retaining memories but also about ensuring a high quality of life in our later years. Thankfully, there are numerous strategies available to promote a healthy brain and offset age-related cognitive decline. By incorporating these practices into our daily routines, we can optimize brain function and embrace the aging process with vigor and purpose.

Social connection is another crucial aspect of brain health. Maintaining strong social ties with friends, family, and community members provides cognitive stimulation, emotional support, and a sense of belonging—all vital for healthy aging. Engage in meaningful social activities, cultivate supportive relationships, and prioritize spending time with loved ones to support brain health and overall well-being.

Continuously challenging the brain with new experiences and learning opportunities is also beneficial for cognitive health. Taking up hobbies, pursuing interests, and exploring unfamiliar subjects can stimulate neural pathways and enhance cognitive reserve. By embracing lifelong learning and seeking out novel experiences, we can build resilience against cognitive decline and age-related cognitive challenges.

Prioritizing brain health is essential for maintaining cognitive vitality and quality of life as we age. By incorporating strategies such as staying mentally active, maintaining a balanced diet, engaging in regular physical exercise, getting quality sleep, managing stress effectively, staying socially connected, and challenging our brains with new experiences, we can optimize brain function and embrace the aging process with vitality and purpose.

Furthermore, emerging research suggests that certain lifestyle factors, such as cognitive engagement, diet, exercise, sleep, stress management, social interaction, and continuous learning, can profoundly impact brain health and resilience against cognitive decline. These factors, when integrated into a holistic approach to wellness, offer a comprehensive strategy for promoting cognitive vitality and supporting healthy aging.

Cognitive engagement goes beyond mere mental stimulation; it encompasses the active pursuit of activities that challenge and stimulate the brain. Engaging in cognitive activities that require problem-solving, critical thinking, and creativity can help build cognitive reserve—a form of protection against age-related cognitive decline. Moreover, lifelong learning fosters cognitive flexibility, adaptability, and resilience, allowing individuals to navigate cognitive challenges more effectively as they age.

Dietary choices play a significant role in brain health and cognitive function. Research indicates that certain nutrients, such as omega-3 fatty acids, antioxidants, vitamins, and minerals, have neuroprotective effects and can support cognitive function throughout the lifespan. Incorporating a variety of nutrient-rich foods into the diet, including leafy greens, fatty fish, berries, nuts, and seeds, can provide the essential building blocks for optimal brain health and function.

Regular physical exercise has been shown to exert beneficial effects on brain structure and function. Aerobic exercise, in particular, has been associated with improvements in cognitive performance, memory, and executive function. Additionally, strength training and flexibility exercises can enhance overall physical health and contribute to cognitive well-being. The cumulative effects of regular exercise extend beyond physical fitness to encompass cognitive resilience and emotional well-being.

Quality sleep is fundamental for brain health and cognitive function. During sleep, the brain undergoes essential processes involved in memory consolidation, synaptic pruning, and neural repair. Disrupted or inadequate sleep can impair cognitive performance, mood regulation, and overall brain health. Therefore, prioritizing sleep hygiene practices and establishing a consistent sleep routine are critical for maintaining optimal brain function and cognitive vitality.

Effective stress management is essential for protecting brain health and mitigating the negative effects of chronic stress on cognitive function. Chronic stress has been linked to structural and functional changes in the brain, including hippocampal atrophy and impaired synaptic plasticity. By adopting stress-reduction techniques such as mindfulness meditation, relaxation exercises, and stress-reducing activities, individuals can cultivate resilience and promote brain health throughout the aging process.

Social interaction and meaningful connections play a vital role in cognitive health and emotional well-being. Engaging in social activities, maintaining friendships, and participating in community events provide opportunities for cognitive stimulation, emotional support, and a sense of belonging. Research suggests that social isolation and loneliness are associated with increased risk of cognitive decline and dementia, highlighting the importance of staying socially connected as we age.

Incorporating cognitive challenges into everyday life is crucial for maintaining cognitive vitality and promoting brain health. Whether it's learning a new language, mastering a musical instrument, or tackling a complex puzzle, engaging in intellectually stimulating activities can help preserve cognitive function and enhance overall well-being. By embracing a mindset of lifelong learning and intellectual curiosity, individuals can cultivate cognitive resilience and thrive as they age.

Promoting brain health and cognitive vitality requires a multifaceted approach that addresses various lifestyle factors, including cognitive engagement, diet, exercise, sleep, stress management, social interaction, and continuous learning. By incorporating these strategies into our daily lives, we can optimize brain function, enhance cognitive resilience, and embrace the aging process with vitality and purpose.

Moreover, recent advancements in neuroscience have underscored the importance of neuroplasticity—the brain's ability to reorganize and form new neural connections in response to experience and learning. This remarkable capacity for adaptation means that the brain remains malleable throughout life, offering opportunities for growth and development even in later years. By actively engaging in cognitive activities and challenging the mind, individuals can harness the power of neuroplasticity to promote cognitive vitality and offset age-related decline.

The role of lifestyle factors in brain health extends beyond individual behaviors to encompass broader environmental influences. Factors such as socioeconomic status, education level, access to healthcare, and community resources can profoundly impact cognitive health and resilience. Addressing disparities in access to educational and healthcare resources is essential for promoting equitable opportunities for brain health across diverse populations.

Furthermore, emerging research suggests that certain habits and behaviors may exert neuroprotective effects and reduce the risk of cognitive decline and dementia. For example, regular engagement in intellectually stimulating activities has been associated with a lower risk of cognitive impairment in later life. Similarly, adherence to a Mediterranean-style diet, characterized by high consumption of fruits, vegetables, whole grains, and olive oil, has been linked to better cognitive function and a reduced risk of cognitive decline.

Physical activity not only benefits brain health but also plays a crucial role in maintaining overall health and well-being as we age. In addition to its cognitive benefits, regular exercise has been shown to reduce the risk of chronic conditions such as cardiovascular disease, diabetes, and obesity—all of which are risk factors for cognitive decline. Therefore, promoting physical activity at both the individual and community levels is essential for supporting healthy aging and preserving cognitive function.

The importance of early intervention and prevention strategies cannot be overstated when it comes to promoting brain health and reducing the burden of age-related cognitive decline. By implementing evidence-based interventions aimed at optimizing cognitive function and reducing modifiable risk factors, policymakers, healthcare providers, and community stakeholders can help empower individuals to age successfully and maintain their cognitive vitality.

Moreover, fostering a culture of lifelong learning and intellectual curiosity is essential for promoting brain health across the lifespan. Educational initiatives aimed at promoting cognitive stimulation and providing opportunities for continued learning can help individuals build cognitive reserve and resilience against age-related cognitive decline. By investing in educational programs and resources that support cognitive health, societies can empower individuals to thrive intellectually and maintain their cognitive abilities as they age.

Promoting brain health and cognitive vitality requires a comprehensive approach that addresses individual behaviors, environmental influences, and societal factors. By incorporating strategies such as cognitive engagement, healthy lifestyle choices, early intervention, and lifelong learning, we can optimize brain function, reduce the risk of cognitive decline, and enhance overall well-being as we age. Together, we can build a future where cognitive vitality is valued, protected, and preserved for all individuals, regardless of age or background.

Furthermore, advances in technology offer promising avenues for promoting brain health and cognitive vitality. Digital cognitive training programs, virtual reality interventions, and brain-computer interface technologies have emerged as innovative tools for enhancing cognitive function and supporting healthy aging. These technologies provide personalized and engaging experiences that target specific cognitive domains, such as memory, attention, and executive function, and can be tailored to individual needs and preferences.

Moreover, promoting brain health requires a holistic approach that recognizes the interconnectedness of physical, mental, and emotional well-being. Integrative practices such as yoga, tai chi, and mindfulness-based interventions offer additional avenues for supporting cognitive health and resilience. These practices not only promote relaxation and stress reduction but also enhance cognitive function, emotional regulation, and overall brain health.

Furthermore, promoting brain health necessitates collaboration across disciplines and sectors to address the complex and multifaceted nature of cognitive aging. By fostering partnerships between researchers, healthcare professionals, policymakers, educators, and community organizations, we can develop comprehensive strategies that promote brain health and cognitive vitality at individual, community, and societal levels.

Moreover, promoting brain health requires a shift in societal attitudes and perceptions towards aging and cognitive function. By challenging ageist stereotypes and promoting a positive view of aging, we can create environments that support cognitive health and well-being across the lifespan. Encouraging intergenerational connections, promoting age-friendly communities, and celebrating the contributions of older adults can help foster a culture of inclusion, respect, and support for cognitive aging.

Furthermore, promoting brain health involves addressing disparities in access to resources and opportunities that impact cognitive function and well-being. Socioeconomic factors, such as income, education, and social support, can influence cognitive health outcomes and contribute to disparities in cognitive aging. Therefore, efforts to promote brain health must prioritize equity and social justice to ensure that all individuals have the opportunity to age with dignity and maintain their cognitive vitality.

Promoting brain health and cognitive vitality requires a multifaceted and interdisciplinary approach that addresses individual, environmental, and societal factors. By integrating strategies such as technology-based interventions, integrative practices, collaboration across sectors, challenging ageist attitudes, and addressing disparities in access to resources, we can create environments that support cognitive health and well-being for all individuals as they age. Together, we can build a future where cognitive aging is embraced as a natural and valued aspect of the human experience, and where individuals can age with dignity, resilience, and vitality.

Chapter V. Brain-Boosting Activities

Overview of activities that can help improve brain function

The human brain is a complex organ with incredible capabilities. It controls our thoughts, emotions, actions, and every aspect of our lives. Just like any other part of our body, it's essential to keep our brains healthy and functioning optimally. Fortunately, there are various activities and habits that can help improve brain function and overall cognitive health.

One of the most effective ways to enhance brain function is through regular physical exercise. Exercise not only benefits the body but also the mind. Research has shown that aerobic exercise, such as walking, jogging, or cycling, can increase the size of the hippocampus, the part of the brain responsible for memory and learning. Exercise also promotes the release of chemicals called neurotransmitters, which help improve mood and cognitive function.

In addition to physical exercise, mental stimulation is crucial for maintaining brain health. Engaging in activities that challenge the mind, such as puzzles, crosswords, or learning a new skill, can help keep the brain sharp and improve cognitive function. These activities stimulate the brain's neural pathways, promoting the growth of new connections and improving overall brain function.

Furthermore, maintaining a healthy diet is essential for brain health. Consuming a diet rich in fruits, vegetables, whole grains, and healthy fats provides essential nutrients that support brain function. Omega-3 fatty acids, found in fish, nuts, and seeds, are particularly beneficial for brain health, as they help reduce inflammation and promote the growth of new brain cells.

Adequate sleep is another critical factor in maintaining brain health. During sleep, the brain consolidates memories and processes information, essential for learning and cognitive function. Chronic sleep deprivation can impair cognitive function, memory, and mood, so it's important to prioritize getting enough quality sleep each night.

Managing stress is also essential for brain health. Chronic stress can have detrimental effects on the brain, impairing memory, attention, and decision-making skills. Practicing relaxation techniques such as meditation, deep breathing, or yoga can help reduce stress and promote brain health.

Lastly, staying socially engaged and maintaining strong social connections is vital for brain health. Social interaction stimulates the brain and helps ward off feelings of loneliness and isolation, which can have negative effects on cognitive function. Engaging in activities with friends and loved ones, volunteering, or joining clubs or social groups can help keep the brain active and healthy.

There are many activities and habits that can help improve brain function and overall cognitive health. By incorporating regular physical exercise, mental stimulation, a healthy diet, adequate sleep, stress management techniques, and social engagement into your daily routine, you can help keep your brain sharp and functioning at its best for years to come.

The human brain, a marvel of complexity, orchestrates our every thought, emotion, and action. Nurturing this vital organ is paramount, akin to caring for any other part of our body. Fortunately, an array of activities and habits exists to bolster brain function and fortify cognitive vitality.

In summation, a myriad of practices and habits converge to enhance brain function and uphold cognitive well-being. Embracing regular physical exercise, mental stimulation, a nutrient-rich diet, sufficient sleep, stress management strategies, and robust social engagement fosters enduring cognitive vitality. By integrating these elements into daily routines, individuals can cultivate brain health, ensuring optimal function and resilience across the lifespan.

Moreover, emerging research sheds light on the symbiotic relationship between gut health and brain function. The gut-brain axis, a bidirectional communication network, underscores the profound impact of gut microbiota on cognitive processes. Consuming a diverse array of probiotic-rich foods, such as yogurt, kefir, and fermented vegetables, fosters a flourishing gut microbiome, thereby enhancing cognitive resilience.

Cognitive enrichment extends beyond solitary pursuits to encompass the realm of interpersonal dynamics. Collaborative endeavors, group problem-solving activities, and team-based projects invigorate cognitive faculties, fostering creativity and resilience. Harnessing the collective wisdom of diverse perspectives amplifies cognitive insights, propelling innovation and adaptive thinking.

Furthermore, embracing a lifelong learning ethos confers profound benefits for brain health and cognitive longevity. Cultivating intellectual curiosity, pursuing continuing education opportunities, and exploring new domains of knowledge stimulate neuroplasticity, fortifying cognitive reserves against age-related decline. Adopting a growth mindset, characterized by resilience and a penchant for embracing challenges, nurtures cognitive flexibility and adaptive learning strategies.

Incorporating mindfulness practices into daily routines fosters cognitive equilibrium and emotional well-being. Mindfulness meditation, characterized by non-judgmental awareness and focused attention, cultivates emotional resilience and cognitive clarity. By fostering present-moment awareness, mindfulness techniques mitigate rumination and anxiety, fostering cognitive clarity and emotional balance.

Moreover, leveraging technology as a tool for cognitive enhancement holds promise in the contemporary digital age. Brain-training apps, cognitive games, and virtual reality simulations offer engaging platforms for honing cognitive skills and fostering neuroplasticity. Integrating technology-assisted interventions into cognitive wellness regimens augments traditional approaches, catering to diverse learning styles and preferences.

In essence, the pursuit of cognitive wellness transcends individual habits to encompass holistic lifestyle choices and environmental factors. Cultivating a supportive ecosystem that nurtures cognitive health entails fostering a balanced interplay of physical, mental, social, and emotional well-being. By embracing a multifaceted approach to cognitive wellness, individuals can unlock their full cognitive potential, fostering resilience and vitality across the lifespan.

Furthermore, the integration of art and creativity into daily life serves as a potent catalyst for cognitive enrichment. Engaging in artistic pursuits, such as painting, sculpting, or playing a musical instrument, stimulates neural networks associated with creativity and innovation. The act of creation fosters cognitive flexibility, encouraging novel approaches to problem-solving and enhancing emotional expression.

Embracing nature as a source of cognitive rejuvenation offers myriad benefits for brain health and well-being. Spending time outdoors, whether hiking through lush forests or strolling along sun-kissed beaches, confers cognitive respite from the demands of modern life. Nature immersion fosters mindfulness and sensory engagement, revitalizing cognitive faculties and reducing stress levels.

Moreover, fostering a sense of purpose and meaning in life contributes profoundly to cognitive resilience and emotional well-being. Engaging in activities aligned with personal values and aspirations instills a sense of fulfillment and satisfaction, bolstering psychological resilience. Cultivating meaningful connections with others and contributing to the greater good imbues life with purpose, fostering cognitive vitality and emotional equilibrium.

Incorporating mindfulness-based practices into everyday activities cultivates cognitive presence and emotional resilience. Mindful eating, characterized by attentiveness to sensory experiences and appreciation of nourishing foods, fosters a healthy relationship with food and promotes cognitive clarity. Similarly, mindful communication and interpersonal interactions deepen connections with others, fostering empathy and emotional intelligence.

Furthermore, nurturing a restorative sleep environment is essential for optimizing cognitive function and overall well-being. Creating a sleep sanctuary conducive to relaxation and rejuvenation, characterized by dim lighting, comfortable bedding, and a soothing ambiance, promotes restful sleep. Prioritizing consistent sleep schedules and implementing pre-sleep rituals, such as reading or practicing relaxation techniques, facilitates the transition to restorative slumber.

Additionally, embracing cognitive challenges and embracing novelty fosters cognitive resilience and adaptive learning. Engaging in activities that push the boundaries of one's comfort zone, such as learning a new language, mastering a musical instrument, or tackling complex puzzles, stimulates neuroplasticity and enhances cognitive agility. Embracing lifelong learning as a cornerstone of cognitive wellness fosters intellectual curiosity and a zest for exploration.

Fostering cognitive wellness encompasses a multifaceted approach that integrates diverse strategies and practices. By embracing creativity, nature, purpose, mindfulness, restorative sleep, and cognitive challenges, individuals can cultivate robust cognitive health and emotional well-being. Embracing a holistic lifestyle that nurtures cognitive vitality empowers individuals to thrive intellectually and emotionally, fostering resilience and fulfillment across the lifespan.

Furthermore, the exploration of cultural activities and exposure to diverse experiences serve as enriching stimuli for cognitive vitality. Attending cultural events, such as art exhibitions, theater performances, or music concerts, broadens cognitive horizons and fosters appreciation for different perspectives. Exposure to diverse cultural expressions nurtures cognitive flexibility and empathy, enriching one's understanding of the world.

Embracing reflective practices, such as journaling or contemplative walks, promotes introspection and self-awareness, fostering cognitive clarity and emotional resilience. Taking time for introspection allows individuals to process experiences, clarify values, and cultivate a deeper understanding of themselves and others. Reflective practices nurture cognitive flexibility, empowering individuals to navigate life's complexities with greater insight and equanimity.

Moreover, fostering a sense of community and belonging contributes to cognitive well-being and psychological flourishing. Participating in community activities, volunteering, or joining social groups cultivates social connections and support networks, buffering against loneliness and isolation. Strong social ties foster a sense of belonging and purpose, enhancing cognitive resilience and emotional well-being.

Additionally, embracing the arts as a form of self-expression and emotional regulation offers therapeutic benefits for cognitive health. Engaging in creative pursuits, such as writing, painting, or dancing, provides an outlet for processing emotions and channeling creative energy. Artistic expression fosters emotional catharsis and self-discovery, promoting cognitive integration and emotional well-being.

Furthermore, incorporating mindfulness-based interventions into therapeutic practices offers effective strategies for enhancing cognitive resilience and emotional regulation. Mindfulness-based cognitive therapy (MBCT) integrates mindfulness practices with cognitive-behavioral techniques to alleviate symptoms of depression, anxiety, and stress. Cultivating present-moment awareness and non-judgmental acceptance fosters emotional resilience and cognitive flexibility, empowering individuals to navigate life's challenges with greater equanimity.

Moreover, engaging in meaningful leisure activities that align with personal interests and values fosters cognitive engagement and emotional fulfillment. Pursuing hobbies, interests, or creative pursuits promotes a sense of accomplishment and joy, enhancing cognitive well-being and overall quality of life. By prioritizing leisure activities that nourish the mind and soul, individuals cultivate resilience and vitality in the face of life's challenges.

Fostering cognitive wellness encompasses a holistic approach that integrates diverse practices and experiences. By embracing cultural enrichment, reflective practices, community engagement, artistic expression, mindfulness interventions, and meaningful leisure activities, individuals can cultivate robust cognitive health and emotional well-being. Nurturing cognitive vitality empowers individuals to lead fulfilling lives characterized by resilience, creativity, and emotional flourishing.

Cognitive exercises and mental challenges for older adults

As we age, it's natural for cognitive function to decline to some extent. However, there are many ways older adults can maintain and even improve their cognitive abilities through cognitive exercises and mental challenges.

One of the most effective cognitive exercises for older adults is memory training. Memory exercises can help improve both short-term and long-term memory, making it easier to recall names, dates, and other important information. Simple memory games such as matching games, word recall exercises, and puzzles can help keep the mind sharp and improve memory function.

In addition to memory training, older adults can benefit from activities that challenge other cognitive skills, such as attention, problem-solving, and reasoning. Crossword puzzles, Sudoku, and other brain teasers are excellent ways to stimulate the mind and improve cognitive function. Learning a new skill or hobby, such as playing a musical instrument or learning a new language, can also provide a mental challenge and help keep the brain active and engaged.

Furthermore, social interaction is essential for maintaining cognitive function in older adults. Engaging in conversations, participating in group activities, and spending time with friends and family can help stimulate the brain and ward off feelings of loneliness and isolation, which can contribute to cognitive decline.

Physical exercise is also important for brain health in older adults. Exercise increases blood flow to the brain, promoting the growth of new brain cells and improving cognitive function. Activities such as walking, swimming, or tai chi are excellent options for older adults, as they are low-impact and can be easily adapted to individual fitness levels.

In addition to these cognitive exercises and mental challenges, it's important for older adults to maintain a healthy lifestyle overall. Eating a balanced diet rich in fruits, vegetables, whole grains, and lean protein can provide essential nutrients that support brain health. Getting enough quality sleep each night is also crucial for cognitive function, as sleep helps consolidate memories and process information.

Cognitive exercises and mental challenges are essential for maintaining and improving cognitive function in older adults. By incorporating memory training, brain teasers, social interaction, physical exercise, and a healthy lifestyle into their daily routine, older adults can keep their minds sharp and functioning at their best as they age.

As individuals progress through life, it's common for cognitive abilities to undergo changes. These alterations, though part of the natural aging process, can be managed effectively through various cognitive exercises and mental engagements tailored for older adults.

In essence, the integration of cognitive exercises and mental engagements into the daily regimen is indispensable for sustaining and enhancing cognitive function among older adults. By embracing memory training, brain-stimulating activities, social interaction, physical exercise, and a health-conscious lifestyle, seniors can fortify their mental acuity and navigate the aging process with resilience and vigor.

Furthermore, emerging research underscores the importance of maintaining an intellectually stimulating environment for older adults. Exposure to novel experiences, such as visiting museums, attending lectures, or engaging in intellectual discussions, can provide continuous cognitive enrichment and contribute to cognitive resilience over time.

Technology also offers a wealth of opportunities for cognitive engagement among seniors. Learning to use smartphones, tablets, or computers not only provides mental stimulation but also fosters connectivity with loved ones through social media platforms or video calls. Additionally, there is a plethora of brain-training apps and online resources designed specifically to challenge and enhance various cognitive functions.

Moreover, engaging in mindfulness practices such as meditation or yoga can yield significant cognitive benefits for older adults. These practices promote relaxation, reduce stress, and enhance attention and concentration—all of which are vital components of cognitive well-being. Regular mindfulness exercises can also help older individuals manage age-related cognitive changes more effectively.

Another crucial aspect often overlooked is the importance of maintaining a sense of purpose and meaning in life. Older adults who remain actively engaged in meaningful pursuits, whether through volunteering, pursuing hobbies, or setting personal goals, tend to exhibit better cognitive function and overall well-being. Cultivating a sense of purpose not only provides motivation but also stimulates cognitive processes by keeping the mind focused and stimulated.

Furthermore, it's essential to recognize that cognitive abilities can vary widely among older adults due to factors such as genetics, lifestyle, and overall health. Therefore, personalized approaches to cognitive maintenance and enhancement are key. Individuals should tailor their cognitive exercises and activities to their specific strengths, interests, and abilities, ensuring that they derive maximum benefit from their efforts.

Fostering a supportive and encouraging environment is crucial for older adults embarking on a journey to maintain and improve their cognitive function. Family members, caregivers, and healthcare professionals play pivotal roles in providing encouragement, assistance, and resources to help seniors stay mentally active and engaged. By fostering a culture of lifelong learning and cognitive wellness, society can empower older adults to age gracefully and maintain optimal cognitive health well into their later years.

Additionally, ongoing research emphasizes the significance of maintaining social connections and community engagement in supporting cognitive health among older adults. Participation in social groups, clubs, or community centers not only provides opportunities for social interaction but also encourages mental stimulation through shared activities and discussions. These social bonds can serve as a protective factor against cognitive decline by fostering a sense of belonging and purpose.

Furthermore, incorporating relaxation techniques and stress management strategies into daily life can contribute to cognitive well-being in older adults. High levels of chronic stress have been linked to cognitive impairment and an increased risk of dementia. Therefore, practices such as deep breathing exercises, progressive muscle relaxation, or guided imagery can help seniors alleviate stress and promote mental clarity.

Moreover, maintaining an active and intellectually curious mindset is crucial for preserving cognitive function as individuals age. Continuously seeking out new challenges, setting goals, and embracing lifelong learning can help older adults stay mentally agile and adaptable. Whether it's enrolling in classes, attending workshops, or pursuing creative endeavors, the pursuit of intellectual growth can be a powerful antidote to cognitive stagnation.

Another important consideration is the role of regular cognitive assessments and monitoring in identifying early signs of cognitive decline or impairment. By staying vigilant and proactive about cognitive health, older adults and their healthcare providers can intervene early with targeted interventions or treatments to mitigate the progression of cognitive decline.

Furthermore, it's essential to recognize that maintaining cognitive health is not solely an individual responsibility but also a societal one. Communities, businesses, and policymakers can contribute to creating age-friendly environments that promote cognitive well-being through initiatives such as accessible public spaces, lifelong learning programs, and policies that support healthy aging.

Preserving and enhancing cognitive function among older adults requires a multifaceted approach that encompasses cognitive exercises, social engagement, stress management, lifelong learning, and community support. By embracing these strategies and fostering a culture of cognitive wellness, individuals can optimize their cognitive health and quality of life as they age.

Furthermore, it's important to acknowledge the impact of mental health on cognitive function in older adults. Conditions such as depression and anxiety can significantly impair cognitive abilities and exacerbate age-related cognitive decline. Therefore, prioritizing mental health and seeking support when needed is essential for maintaining cognitive well-being. Therapeutic interventions, such as cognitive-behavioral therapy or counseling, can help older adults address underlying mental health issues and improve overall cognitive function.

Additionally, staying intellectually engaged through reading, writing, or engaging in intellectually stimulating conversations can provide ongoing cognitive stimulation for older adults. These activities not only keep the mind active but also promote cognitive flexibility and creativity, which are important aspects of cognitive health.

Furthermore, maintaining a healthy balance between mental and physical activities is crucial for overall well-being. While cognitive exercises are important, they should be complemented by regular physical activity to support brain health. Engaging in activities that promote cardiovascular health, such as aerobic exercise or strength training, can have positive effects on cognitive function by increasing blood flow to the brain and promoting the release of neurotrophic factors that support brain plasticity.

Moreover, fostering a supportive and inclusive environment for older adults is essential for promoting cognitive health and well-being. Ageism and stereotypes about cognitive decline can have negative effects on older adults' self-perception and mental health. Therefore, creating age-friendly communities that value and respect the contributions of older adults can help combat age-related stigma and promote positive attitudes towards aging and cognitive health.

Lastly, embracing a proactive approach to brain health by adopting healthy lifestyle habits early in life can have long-lasting benefits for cognitive function in older adulthood. Prioritizing factors such as diet, exercise, sleep, and mental stimulation throughout the lifespan can help build cognitive reserve and reduce the risk of cognitive decline later in life.

Maintaining cognitive health in older adulthood requires a comprehensive approach that addresses the interplay between physical, mental, and social factors. By incorporating strategies to promote mental well-being, engage in intellectually stimulating activities, prioritize physical health, and create supportive environments, older adults can optimize their cognitive function and overall quality of life as they age.

Furthermore, recent studies have highlighted the potential benefits of incorporating technology-based interventions into cognitive health strategies for older adults. Digital platforms, including smartphone apps, virtual reality programs, and online cognitive training tools, offer convenient and accessible ways to engage in brain-stimulating activities from the comfort of home. These technologies can provide personalized cognitive exercises, track progress over time, and offer real-time feedback, enhancing motivation and adherence to cognitive training regimens.

Additionally, promoting cognitive diversity and inclusivity is essential for ensuring that cognitive health strategies meet the needs of diverse older adult populations. This includes tailoring interventions to accommodate individuals with varying cultural backgrounds, linguistic abilities, and cognitive profiles. By embracing diversity and cultural sensitivity in cognitive health programming, healthcare providers and policymakers can better address the unique needs and preferences of older adults from diverse communities.

Moreover, integrating cognitive health promotion into existing healthcare systems can enhance access to services and support for older adults. This includes incorporating cognitive screenings into routine healthcare visits, providing education and resources on cognitive health management, and facilitating referrals to specialized services when needed. By embedding cognitive health promotion within primary care settings, healthcare providers can identify cognitive issues early and intervene promptly to optimize outcomes for older adults.

Furthermore, fostering intergenerational connections and interactions can promote cognitive health and well-being for older adults. Intergenerational programs that bring together older adults and younger generations for shared activities, mentorship opportunities, or intergenerational learning experiences can provide valuable social engagement and cognitive stimulation for older adults. These programs also offer opportunities for knowledge exchange, skill development, and mutual support across age groups, fostering a sense of community and belonging for participants of all ages.

Lastly, advancing research in the field of cognitive aging is essential for developing evidence-based interventions and strategies to support cognitive health in older adults. By investing in research on cognitive training, lifestyle interventions, brain health biomarkers, and novel therapies, scientists can better understand the mechanisms underlying age-related cognitive decline and identify new approaches to prevention and treatment. This research can inform the development of targeted interventions to promote cognitive resilience, delay the onset of cognitive impairment, and improve quality of life for older adults.

Promoting cognitive health and well-being in older adulthood requires a multifaceted approach that addresses individual, social, cultural, and systemic factors. By integrating technology-based interventions, promoting cognitive diversity and inclusivity, embedding cognitive health promotion within healthcare systems, fostering intergenerational connections, and advancing research in the field, stakeholders can work together to optimize cognitive function and enhance quality of life for older adults as they age.

Benefits of social engagement and lifelong learning on brain health

Social engagement and lifelong learning are two key factors that can have significant benefits for brain health. Both activities stimulate the brain, promote the growth of new neural connections, and help ward off cognitive decline.

One of the primary benefits of social engagement on brain health is its ability to reduce feelings of loneliness and isolation, which are known risk factors for cognitive decline and dementia. Regular social interaction stimulates the brain and helps maintain cognitive function in older adults. Engaging in conversations, participating in group activities, and spending time with friends and family can help keep the mind sharp and improve overall brain health.

Furthermore, social engagement provides opportunities for cognitive stimulation and mental challenges. Engaging in discussions, playing games, and participating in group activities all require the use of cognitive skills such as attention, memory, and problem-solving. These activities help keep the brain active and engaged, promoting the growth of new neural connections and improving cognitive function.

Lifelong learning is another powerful tool for promoting brain health. Learning new skills, acquiring knowledge, and challenging oneself intellectually all provide mental stimulation and help keep the brain sharp. Whether it's learning a new language, taking up a new hobby, or enrolling in a continuing education class, lifelong learning offers countless opportunities for cognitive growth and development.

In addition to stimulating the brain, lifelong learning has been shown to have other positive effects on brain health. Research has found that engaging in intellectually stimulating activities throughout life can help build a cognitive reserve, which may help protect against cognitive decline and dementia in later years. Lifelong learning also promotes a sense of purpose and fulfillment, which are important factors for overall well-being and brain health.

Social engagement and lifelong learning are essential for maintaining and improving brain health. By staying socially active, engaging in intellectually stimulating activities, and continually challenging oneself to learn and grow, individuals can keep their minds sharp and functioning at their best throughout life.

Social engagement and lifelong learning are not just enjoyable pastimes; they are essential ingredients for maintaining optimal brain health and function, especially as we age. These two factors are deeply intertwined, offering a myriad of benefits that extend far beyond mere enjoyment.

Let's delve into the significance of social engagement first. Beyond its role in fostering connections and relationships, social interaction plays a crucial role in brain health. Loneliness and isolation, increasingly prevalent in modern society, pose significant risks to cognitive function. Research has established a clear link between social isolation and cognitive decline, making regular social engagement a powerful antidote. By participating in conversations, group activities, and spending time with loved ones, individuals stimulate their brains, keeping cognitive abilities sharp and intact.

Moreover, social engagement isn't merely about companionship; it serves as a platform for cognitive stimulation. Engaging in discussions, playing games, or tackling group activities all demand cognitive skills such as attention, memory, and problem-solving. These mental exercises help keep the brain agile and promote the formation of new neural connections, crucial for maintaining cognitive function.

On the other hand, lifelong learning stands as another pillar of brain health. The act of acquiring new knowledge, skills, and experiences throughout life provides continuous mental stimulation, keeping the brain agile and adaptable. Whether it's mastering a new language, delving into a new hobby, or enrolling in educational courses, lifelong learning offers endless opportunities for cognitive growth.

Beyond mental stimulation, lifelong learning has far-reaching benefits for brain health. Studies indicate that engaging in intellectually challenging activities can build a cognitive reserve, essentially a buffer against cognitive decline and dementia in later life. This cognitive reserve acts as a safeguard, allowing individuals to maintain cognitive function despite the brain changes associated with aging.

Furthermore, lifelong learning fosters a sense of purpose and fulfillment, crucial components of overall well-being. Pursuing intellectual endeavors gives individuals a reason to wake up excited each day, fueling motivation and enthusiasm for life. This sense of purpose has profound effects on mental health, contributing to lower stress levels and improved overall cognitive function.

Social engagement and lifelong learning are indispensable for nurturing and enhancing brain health throughout life. By prioritizing social interactions and embracing opportunities for continuous learning, individuals can safeguard their cognitive abilities and enjoy a fulfilling and vibrant existence well into old age.

Moreover, the benefits of social engagement and lifelong learning extend beyond individual well-being to encompass broader societal impacts. Communities enriched with vibrant social networks and accessible learning opportunities tend to experience lower rates of cognitive decline and enhanced overall quality of life for residents of all ages. By fostering environments that encourage social interaction and lifelong learning, societies can promote healthier aging and reduce the burden of age-related cognitive disorders on healthcare systems and families.

Additionally, emerging research suggests that the benefits of social engagement and lifelong learning may extend to physical health as well. Studies have found correlations between strong social connections, active lifestyles, and better cardiovascular health, which, in turn, can positively influence brain function. Similarly, engaging in regular physical activity, often facilitated by social interactions and participation in group activities, has been linked to improved cognitive function and reduced risk of cognitive decline.

Furthermore, the integration of technology into social engagement and lifelong learning initiatives has opened up new avenues for accessibility and inclusivity. Online communities, virtual learning platforms, and digital resources offer individuals of all ages opportunities to connect, learn, and engage in intellectually stimulating activities from the comfort of their homes. Leveraging technology in this manner not only broadens access to social and educational resources but also facilitates intergenerational connections, as older adults can interact with younger generations in virtual spaces, exchanging knowledge and experiences.

Despite the myriad benefits, challenges persist in ensuring equitable access to social engagement and lifelong learning opportunities for all individuals. Socioeconomic disparities, geographic barriers, and digital divides can limit access to these enriching experiences, particularly among marginalized communities and older adults living in rural or underserved areas. Addressing these challenges requires a multifaceted approach, involving community partnerships, policy initiatives, and technological innovation to create inclusive environments where everyone can thrive.

Social engagement and lifelong learning are dynamic processes that play integral roles in maintaining brain health, fostering personal fulfillment, and enriching communities. By embracing opportunities for social interaction, intellectual growth, and continued learning, individuals can cultivate resilience against cognitive decline and enhance their overall quality of life. Moreover, by addressing barriers to access and promoting inclusivity, societies can ensure that everyone has the opportunity to age with dignity, vitality, and purpose.

Furthermore, the intersection of social engagement and lifelong learning holds promise for addressing broader societal challenges, such as ageism and social isolation. By creating intergenerational spaces that encourage knowledge exchange and mutual support, communities can foster greater understanding and appreciation for individuals of all ages. Intergenerational programs, where older adults mentor younger generations or collaborate on projects, not only provide valuable learning experiences but also challenge stereotypes and promote empathy across age groups.

Moreover, businesses and organizations are recognizing the value of investing in initiatives that promote social engagement and lifelong learning among their employees. Workplace programs that encourage social interaction, offer opportunities for skill development, and support ongoing learning contribute to employee well-being, job satisfaction, and productivity. Recognizing that engaged and fulfilled employees are key assets, companies are increasingly implementing policies and benefits that prioritize personal growth and professional development throughout employees' careers.

Additionally, the benefits of social engagement and lifelong learning extend to mental health outcomes, with research suggesting correlations between active social networks, ongoing learning, and reduced risk of depression and anxiety. Meaningful social connections provide emotional support, buffer against stress, and promote a sense of belonging—all of which are vital for mental well-being. Similarly, the intellectual stimulation derived from lifelong learning can serve as a form of cognitive therapy, offering individuals a sense of purpose and accomplishment that enhances overall psychological resilience.

Furthermore, fostering a culture of curiosity and exploration through social engagement and lifelong learning can have ripple effects throughout society. Individuals who embrace learning as a lifelong pursuit often become advocates for education, inspiring others to seek out new experiences and pursue their passions. Whether through volunteering, mentoring, or community leadership roles, lifelong learners contribute their knowledge and skills to the betterment of society, creating a ripple effect of positive change that extends far beyond themselves.

The symbiotic relationship between social engagement and lifelong learning is a powerful force for personal growth, community vitality, and societal resilience. By embracing opportunities for connection, intellectual enrichment, and personal development, individuals can nurture their minds, bodies, and spirits throughout life's journey. Moreover, by fostering inclusive environments that prioritize access to social and educational resources for all, societies can unlock the full potential of every individual and create a more vibrant and equitable world for generations to come.

Moreover, the benefits of integrating social engagement and lifelong learning extend to fostering creativity and innovation within society. By encouraging individuals to explore new ideas, collaborate with diverse peers, and challenge conventional thinking, these practices cultivate an environment conducive to innovation and problem-solving. Interdisciplinary collaborations, often sparked by social interactions and fueled by ongoing learning, have the potential to address complex challenges facing communities, from sustainability issues to healthcare disparities.

Furthermore, the relationship between social engagement, lifelong learning, and cognitive resilience underscores the importance of adopting a holistic approach to brain health. While genetics and age play significant roles in cognitive decline, lifestyle factors such as social connectedness and intellectual stimulation can exert a profound influence on brain function. As such, public health initiatives and healthcare interventions increasingly emphasize the importance of promoting behaviors that support brain health across the lifespan, including regular physical activity, healthy nutrition, stress management, and, notably, social engagement and lifelong learning.

Additionally, the advent of aging populations worldwide underscores the urgency of prioritizing interventions that support healthy aging and mitigate the burden of age-related cognitive disorders. By investing in programs that promote social engagement and lifelong learning, policymakers can proactively address the growing prevalence of dementia and Alzheimer's disease, reducing healthcare costs and improving the quality of life for older adults. From community-based initiatives to national strategies for healthy aging, there is a growing recognition of the integral role that social connections and intellectual pursuits play in promoting cognitive resilience and preserving independence as individuals age.

Chapter VI. The Future of Brain Aging Research

Brain Aging Research: Exploring Current Trends and Advancements

The study of brain aging has garnered significant attention in recent years as researchers strive to unravel the complexities of cognitive decline and neurodegenerative diseases associated with advancing age. In this chapter, we delve into the current trends and advancements shaping this field of research.

Aging is a natural process that affects every organ in the body, including the brain. As individuals grow older, they may experience changes in memory, cognition, and other cognitive functions. Understanding the underlying mechanisms of age-related cognitive decline is crucial for developing effective interventions to promote healthy aging and mitigate the impact of neurodegenerative diseases such as Alzheimer's and Parkinson's.

One of the prominent trends in brain aging research is the focus on identifying biomarkers that can predict cognitive decline and dementia risk. Advances in neuroimaging techniques, such as magnetic resonance imaging (MRI) and positron emission tomography (PET), have enabled researchers to detect structural and functional changes in the aging brain. By studying these biomarkers, scientists hope to develop early diagnostic tools and targeted interventions for individuals at risk of cognitive decline.

Another area of interest is the role of lifestyle factors in brain aging. Research suggests that factors such as diet, exercise, social engagement, and cognitive stimulation can influence cognitive health in older adults. Lifestyle interventions, such as physical exercise programs and cognitive training exercises, have shown promise in preserving cognitive function and reducing the risk of dementia. Furthermore, emerging evidence indicates that certain dietary patterns, such as the Mediterranean diet, may have protective effects against cognitive decline.

Advancements in genetics and molecular biology have also expanded our understanding of the genetic factors contributing to brain aging and neurodegenerative diseases. Genome-wide association studies (GWAS) have identified genetic variants associated with increased dementia risk, providing insights into the biological pathways involved in disease pathogenesis. Furthermore, the development of gene editing technologies, such as CRISPR, holds potential for targeted interventions to modify disease-causing genes and prevent or treat neurodegenerative disorders.

In addition to genetic factors, researchers are investigating the role of environmental and epigenetic influences on brain aging. Epigenetic modifications, such as DNA methylation and histone acetylation, regulate gene expression patterns and may contribute to age-related changes in the brain. Understanding how environmental factors and lifestyle choices interact with the epigenome to influence cognitive aging is an area of active investigation.

The study of brain aging has become increasingly important in recent years as scientists strive to comprehend the complexities of cognitive decline and neurodegenerative diseases associated with growing older. Aging is a natural process affecting every organ in the body, including the brain, leading to changes in memory, cognition, and other cognitive functions. To develop effective interventions for healthy aging and combat diseases like Alzheimer's and Parkinson's, it's crucial to understand the underlying mechanisms of age-related cognitive decline.

Collaboration and interdisciplinary approaches are driving progress in brain aging research. By bringing together experts from diverse fields, researchers can leverage complementary expertise and resources to tackle complex questions about aging and cognition. Collaborative initiatives facilitate data sharing and accelerate discoveries in the field.

Looking ahead, the integration of technology and artificial intelligence (AI) holds promise for advancing our understanding of brain aging and developing personalized interventions. Wearable devices, smartphone apps, and digital health platforms enable continuous monitoring of cognitive function and behavior, providing real-time data for research and clinical purposes. Machine learning algorithms can analyze large-scale datasets to identify patterns and predictors of cognitive decline, paving the way for precision medicine approaches tailored to individual risk profiles.

Brain aging research is a dynamic and rapidly evolving field with profound implications for public health and aging societies. By leveraging technological advancements, interdisciplinary collaborations, and a deeper understanding of the biological mechanisms underlying cognitive aging, researchers are poised to make significant strides in promoting brain health and improving the quality of life for older adults.

Recent advancements in brain aging research have shed light on the intricate processes underlying cognitive decline and neurodegenerative diseases. As our understanding of the aging brain deepens, it becomes increasingly clear that a multifaceted approach is necessary to address the complexities of cognitive aging effectively.

One promising avenue of research involves exploring the role of inflammation in brain aging. Chronic inflammation has been implicated in various age-related conditions, including cognitive decline and neurodegenerative diseases. Understanding the interplay between the immune system and brain health is crucial for developing targeted interventions to mitigate the effects of inflammation on cognitive function.

Moreover, emerging evidence suggests that the gut-brain axis plays a significant role in brain aging. The gut microbiota, a complex community of microorganisms residing in the gastrointestinal tract, has been linked to various aspects of brain health. Dysbiosis, or imbalance in the gut microbiota composition, has been associated with cognitive decline and neuroinflammation. Investigating strategies to modulate the gut microbiota through diet, probiotics, or fecal microbiota transplantation holds promise for promoting brain health in aging individuals.

Another area of interest in brain aging research is the study of neuroplasticity, the brain's ability to reorganize and adapt in response to experiences and environmental changes. While traditionally believed to decline with age, recent studies have demonstrated that neuroplasticity persists throughout the lifespan. Understanding how to harness and enhance neuroplasticity in older adults could offer novel approaches to preserving cognitive function and resilience against age-related cognitive decline.

Furthermore, the impact of sleep on brain aging is a topic of growing interest among researchers. Sleep disturbances are common in older adults and have been linked to cognitive impairment and neurodegenerative diseases. Investigating the mechanisms underlying the relationship between sleep and brain health could lead to novel interventions for promoting healthy aging and preventing cognitive decline.

In addition to biological factors, psychosocial factors also play a significant role in brain aging. Social isolation, depression, and chronic stress have been associated with accelerated cognitive decline and increased risk of dementia. Developing interventions to address psychosocial factors and promote social connectedness and mental well-being could have profound implications for brain health in aging populations.

Moreover, personalized medicine approaches are gaining traction in brain aging research. Recognizing that individuals age differently and have unique genetic, environmental, and lifestyle profiles, personalized interventions tailored to individual needs and risk factors hold promise for optimizing brain health and preventing cognitive decline.

As we delve deeper into the complexities of brain aging, it becomes evident that a holistic approach encompassing biological, psychological, and social factors is essential for promoting healthy aging and preserving cognitive function in older adults. By continuing to advance our understanding of the aging brain through interdisciplinary collaborations, technological innovations, and personalized interventions, we can strive towards a future where aging is synonymous with vitality and cognitive well-being.

Moreover, recent research has highlighted the importance of vascular health in brain aging. Vascular risk factors such as hypertension, diabetes, and hypercholesterolemia have been associated with an increased risk of cognitive decline and dementia. Understanding the mechanisms by which vascular factors impact brain health is crucial for developing interventions to preserve cognitive function in older adults. Strategies aimed at optimizing vascular health, such as lifestyle modifications and pharmacological treatments, hold promise for reducing the burden of age-related cognitive decline.

Additionally, the role of neuroinflammation in brain aging has garnered significant attention in recent years. Chronic low-grade inflammation in the brain, often referred to as "inflammaging," is thought to contribute to the pathogenesis of neurodegenerative diseases. Identifying the triggers and mediators of neuroinflammation and developing interventions to modulate the inflammatory response could offer novel therapeutic avenues for promoting brain health in aging individuals.

Furthermore, the impact of environmental exposures on brain aging is an area of active investigation. Environmental factors such as air pollution, heavy metals, and pesticides have been implicated in cognitive decline and neurodegenerative diseases. Understanding how these environmental toxins affect brain health and identifying strategies to mitigate their effects could have important implications for public health and aging populations.

Moreover, the gut-brain axis has emerged as a promising target for interventions aimed at promoting brain health in aging individuals. Preclinical and clinical studies have shown that dietary interventions, probiotics, and fecal microbiota transplantation can modulate the gut microbiota and improve cognitive function in older adults. Exploring the mechanisms underlying the gut-brain axis and developing strategies to promote a healthy gut microbiota could offer novel approaches to preserving cognitive function with age.

Furthermore, the field of brain aging research is increasingly recognizing the importance of social determinants of health. Socioeconomic status, education level, and access to healthcare have been identified as significant predictors of cognitive function and dementia risk in older adults. Addressing disparities in access to resources and healthcare services could help reduce the burden of cognitive decline and promote brain health in aging populations.

Brain aging is a multifaceted process influenced by a complex interplay of biological, environmental, and social factors. By continuing to advance our understanding of the mechanisms underlying cognitive aging and neurodegenerative diseases, we can develop targeted interventions to promote brain health and improve the quality of life for older adults. Through interdisciplinary collaborations, technological innovations, and personalized approaches, we can work towards a future where aging is characterized by vitality, resilience, and cognitive well-being.

Exploring Promising Areas of Study for Understanding and Combating Age-Related Cognitive Decline

Age-related cognitive decline is a significant public health challenge, with the prevalence of dementia and other neurodegenerative diseases expected to rise dramatically as the global population ages. In this chapter, we examine promising areas of study that hold potential for understanding and combating cognitive decline in older adults.

One area of research garnering considerable attention is the gut-brain axis and its role in cognitive aging. The gut microbiota, a diverse community of microorganisms residing in the gastrointestinal tract, has emerged as a key player in brain health and function. Studies have shown that changes in the composition and diversity of the gut microbiota, known as dysbiosis, may contribute to age-related cognitive decline and neuroinflammation. Understanding how the gut microbiota interacts with the central nervous system (CNS) could lead to novel interventions, such as probiotics and prebiotics, to support cognitive function in aging individuals.

Another promising avenue of investigation is the role of neuroinflammation in cognitive aging and neurodegenerative diseases. Chronic inflammation in the brain, characterized by the activation of microglia and astrocytes, has been implicated in the pathogenesis of Alzheimer's disease and other age-related dementias. Targeting inflammatory pathways with anti-inflammatory drugs or immunomodulatory agents holds potential for slowing disease progression and preserving cognitive function in older adults.

Advances in neuroimaging technology are also facilitating the study of brain networks and connectivity in aging and dementia. Functional magnetic resonance imaging (fMRI) and diffusion tensor imaging (DTI) allow researchers to map neural circuits and identify disruptions in brain connectivity associated with cognitive decline. Resting-state fMRI studies have revealed alterations in functional connectivity patterns in individuals with mild cognitive impairment

(MCI) and Alzheimer's disease, providing insights into the early stages of neurodegeneration.

Furthermore, research into the role of neuroplasticity and cognitive reserve in aging is shedding light on the brain's ability to adapt and reorganize in response to environmental and lifestyle factors. Cognitive reserve refers to the brain's capacity to withstand age-related changes and pathology through compensatory mechanisms, such as synaptic plasticity and neural network reorganization. Strategies to enhance cognitive reserve, such as lifelong learning, cognitive training, and social engagement, may help to preserve cognitive function and resilience in older adults.

Genetic and epigenetic factors continue to be a focus of investigation in understanding cognitive aging and dementia risk. Genome-wide association studies (GWAS) have identified genetic variants associated with increased susceptibility to Alzheimer's disease and related dementias. Epigenetic modifications, such as DNA methylation and histone acetylation, regulate gene expression patterns and may modulate the risk of cognitive decline in response to environmental stimuli.

In addition to traditional pharmacological approaches, researchers are exploring non-pharmacological interventions for promoting brain health and cognitive function in aging populations. Mind-body interventions, such as mindfulness meditation and yoga, have been shown to reduce stress, improve mood, and enhance cognitive performance in older adults. Aerobic exercise interventions have also demonstrated benefits for cognitive function and brain health, possibly through mechanisms involving increased cerebral blood flow and neurogenesis.

Understanding the complex interplay of biological, environmental, and lifestyle factors in cognitive aging is essential for developing effective strategies to prevent and treat age-related cognitive decline and neurodegenerative diseases. By embracing interdisciplinary approaches and leveraging emerging technologies, researchers are poised to make significant advances in promoting brain health and enhancing cognitive resilience in aging populations.

Age-related cognitive decline represents a significant public health challenge, particularly as the global population ages, leading to an expected surge in dementia and other neurodegenerative diseases. To address this pressing issue, researchers are delving into various promising areas of study aimed at unraveling the mysteries behind cognitive decline in older adults.

Unraveling the intricate interplay of biological, environmental, and lifestyle factors in cognitive aging is paramount for developing effective strategies to prevent and treat age-related cognitive decline and neurodegenerative diseases. By embracing interdisciplinary approaches and harnessing emerging technologies, researchers are poised to make significant strides in promoting brain health and enhancing cognitive resilience in aging populations.

Further exploration into the multifaceted realm of cognitive aging reveals the profound impact of lifestyle factors on brain health. Dietary patterns, for instance, have garnered attention for their potential role in influencing cognitive function in older adults. Emerging evidence suggests that adhering to a Mediterranean-style diet, rich in fruits, vegetables, whole grains, fish, and healthy fats like olive oil, may confer protective benefits against cognitive decline and neurodegenerative diseases. Conversely, diets high in saturated fats and refined sugars have been linked to poorer cognitive outcomes and an increased risk of dementia.

Social engagement represents another critical determinant of cognitive health in aging populations. Maintaining robust social connections through activities like volunteering, participating in group events, and spending time with loved ones not only enriches quality of life but also appears to exert a protective effect against cognitive decline. Socially active individuals often exhibit better cognitive function and a reduced risk of developing dementia compared to their more isolated counterparts. The mechanisms underlying this phenomenon likely involve a combination of factors, including cognitive stimulation, emotional support, and enhanced resilience to stress.

Education and cognitive stimulation throughout life are also recognized as influential factors in shaping cognitive reserve and mitigating age-related cognitive decline. Higher levels of education have been consistently associated with better cognitive outcomes in later life, with individuals possessing greater cognitive reserve exhibiting increased resilience against the adverse effects of aging and pathology. Engaging in mentally stimulating activities such as reading, solving puzzles, learning new skills, and pursuing hobbies can further bolster cognitive reserve and contribute to maintaining cognitive function as individuals age.

In addition to individual lifestyle factors, the broader environmental context in which people live plays a crucial role in shaping cognitive health in aging populations. Socioeconomic status, access to healthcare, built environments, and community resources all impact cognitive aging trajectories. Disparities in these environmental factors contribute to inequalities in cognitive health outcomes, with individuals from disadvantaged backgrounds often facing greater cognitive decline and a higher risk of dementia compared to their more affluent counterparts. Addressing these systemic inequities is essential for promoting cognitive health and fostering healthy aging across diverse populations.

Furthermore, emerging evidence suggests a potential link between sleep quality and cognitive function in older adults. Sleep disturbances, including insomnia and sleep apnea, are common among older individuals and have been associated with cognitive impairment and an increased risk of dementia. Adequate sleep duration and quality are essential for optimal brain function, facilitating processes such as memory consolidation, synaptic plasticity, and clearance of neurotoxic waste products. Interventions aimed at improving sleep hygiene and treating sleep disorders may thus represent promising avenues for preserving cognitive health in aging populations.

Beyond individual lifestyle modifications, public health initiatives aimed at promoting cognitive health and dementia prevention are gaining traction. Awareness campaigns, community-based interventions, and policy efforts aimed at promoting healthy behaviors, fostering social connections, and reducing risk factors for cognitive decline are essential components of comprehensive dementia prevention strategies. By targeting modifiable risk factors at the population level, such initiatives have the potential to mitigate the burden of cognitive decline and dementia on society as a whole.

The quest to understand and address age-related cognitive decline encompasses a broad spectrum of factors, ranging from biological mechanisms to environmental influences and lifestyle choices. By embracing a holistic approach that integrates insights from neuroscience, psychology, public health, and social science, researchers and policymakers can develop more effective strategies for promoting cognitive health and enhancing resilience in aging populations. Through concerted efforts at the individual, community, and societal levels, we can work towards a future where aging is characterized by vitality, autonomy, and cognitive well-being for all.

Moreover, emerging research highlights the importance of mental health in the context of cognitive aging. Depression, anxiety, and other mental health disorders commonly co-occur with cognitive impairment in older adults, exacerbating cognitive decline and impairing overall functioning. Addressing mental health needs through psychotherapy, medication, and support services can play a crucial role in preserving cognitive function and enhancing quality of life in aging populations. Integrating mental health screening and treatment into primary care settings and community-based programs can help identify and address these often overlooked aspects of cognitive health in older adults.

Innovations in technology are also revolutionizing approaches to cognitive assessment, monitoring, and intervention in aging populations. Mobile health applications, wearable devices, and telehealth platforms offer novel opportunities for remotely monitoring cognitive function, delivering personalized interventions, and facilitating early detection of cognitive decline. Virtual reality-based cognitive training programs, cognitive rehabilitation apps, and brain-training games are among the digital tools showing promise in promoting cognitive health and functional independence among older adults. Leveraging these technological advancements can help overcome barriers to accessing traditional healthcare services and empower individuals to take an active role in preserving their cognitive well-being.

Furthermore, the role of vascular health in cognitive aging is increasingly recognized as a critical determinant of brain function in older adults. Vascular risk factors such as hypertension, diabetes, obesity, and smoking contribute to the development of vascular cognitive impairment, a condition characterized by cognitive deficits resulting from cerebrovascular disease. Adopting heart-healthy lifestyle habits, including regular physical activity, a balanced diet, smoking cessation, and management of chronic health conditions, is essential for preserving vascular health and reducing the risk of cognitive decline in aging populations. Multidisciplinary interventions targeting both cardiovascular risk factors and cognitive function hold promise for promoting brain health and preventing vascular-related cognitive impairment in older adults.

Moreover, the impact of environmental exposures on cognitive aging is an area of growing interest and concern. Prolonged exposure to air pollution, heavy metals, pesticides, and other environmental toxins has been linked to cognitive deficits, neuroinflammation, and an increased risk of neurodegenerative diseases in older adults. Mitigating exposure to environmental hazards through regulatory measures, urban planning initiatives, and public health campaigns is crucial for protecting cognitive health and reducing the burden of age-related cognitive decline. Additionally, fostering green spaces, promoting sustainable lifestyles, and advocating for environmental justice can contribute to creating environments that support healthy cognitive aging for all individuals.

The importance of personalized approaches to cognitive health and aging is increasingly recognized in research and clinical practice. Recognizing the heterogeneity of aging trajectories and cognitive outcomes among older adults underscores the need for tailored interventions that address individual preferences, strengths, and challenges. Personalized cognitive interventions may involve combining multiple approaches, such as cognitive training, physical exercise, dietary modification, and social engagement, to create holistic and customized plans that optimize cognitive function and well-being for each individual. Integrating personalized medicine principles into dementia care and cognitive health promotion efforts holds promise for enhancing treatment effectiveness and improving outcomes in aging populations.

In sum, the quest to address age-related cognitive decline requires a multifaceted and interdisciplinary approach that considers the complex interplay of biological, environmental, psychological, and social factors. By advancing our understanding of the determinants of cognitive aging and developing innovative strategies for prevention, early detection, and intervention, we can strive to promote cognitive health and well-being across the lifespan. Through collaborative efforts among researchers, healthcare providers, policymakers, and communities, we can work towards a future where aging is characterized by vitality, resilience, and cognitive flourishing for individuals of all ages.

Exploring the Implications of Ongoing Research for Future Treatments and Interventions

The pursuit of effective treatments and interventions for age-related cognitive decline and neurodegenerative diseases is a pressing challenge in healthcare and biomedical research. In this chapter, we explore the implications of ongoing research in brain aging for the development of future therapies and interventions.

One of the key implications of ongoing research is the potential for early detection and intervention in age-related cognitive decline. Advances in biomarker discovery and neuroimaging techniques offer opportunities to identify individuals at risk of cognitive impairment before the onset of clinical symptoms. Biomarkers such as amyloid-beta and tau protein levels in cerebrospinal fluid or imaging markers of brain atrophy and dysfunction can provide valuable insights into the underlying pathology of neurodegenerative diseases. Early detection allows for timely intervention with disease-modifying therapies or lifestyle interventions aimed at preserving cognitive function and delaying disease progression.

Furthermore, ongoing research is shedding light on the heterogeneity of cognitive aging and dementia, highlighting the need for personalized approaches to treatment and care. Not all older adults experience cognitive decline at the same rate or to the same extent, and factors such as genetics, lifestyle, and comorbidities can influence individual risk profiles. Personalized medicine approaches, informed by genetic and biomarker data, aim to tailor treatment strategies to the unique needs and characteristics of each patient. By targeting specific disease pathways or risk factors, personalized interventions may offer greater efficacy and fewer side effects compared to conventional one-size-fits-all approaches.

Another implication of ongoing research is the potential for disease-modifying therapies to halt or slow the progression of neurodegenerative diseases such as Alzheimer's and

Parkinson's. Despite decades of research, there are currently no treatments available that can reverse or stop the underlying neurodegenerative processes. However, recent advances in our understanding of disease mechanisms and therapeutic targets offer hope for the development of novel interventions. Drug candidates targeting amyloid-beta, tau protein, neuroinflammation, and synaptic dysfunction are undergoing clinical trials, with some showing promising results in early-phase studies. Gene therapies, stem cell-based approaches, and neuroprotective agents are also being investigated as potential disease-modifying treatments for neurodegenerative diseases.

In addition to pharmacological interventions, lifestyle modifications and non-pharmacological approaches have the potential to mitigate cognitive decline and enhance brain health in aging populations. Lifestyle interventions such as physical exercise, cognitive training, social engagement, and dietary modifications have been shown to have beneficial effects on cognitive function and may reduce the risk of dementia. Digital health technologies, including smartphone apps, wearable devices, and telemedicine platforms, offer scalable and cost-effective solutions for delivering personalized interventions and monitoring cognitive health remotely.

Furthermore, ongoing research into the gut-brain axis and the role of the microbiome in cognitive aging may lead to novel therapeutic strategies for promoting brain health. Prebiotics, probiotics, and fecal microbiota transplantation are being investigated for their potential to modulate the gut microbiota and improve cognitive function in older adults. Targeting inflammation and oxidative stress pathways with dietary supplements or nutraceuticals may also offer neuroprotective benefits and enhance resilience against age-related cognitive decline.

Collaboration between academia, industry, and government agencies is essential for translating research findings into clinical practice and addressing the unmet needs of patients with age-related cognitive decline. Multidisciplinary consortia and public-private partnerships facilitate the development of innovative therapies, biomarkers, and diagnostic tools for neurodegenerative diseases. Regulatory agencies play a crucial role in ensuring the safety and efficacy of new treatments, while healthcare providers and patient advocacy organizations are instrumental in raising awareness and promoting access to care for individuals affected by cognitive aging and dementia.

Ongoing research in brain aging holds promise for revolutionizing the diagnosis, treatment, and management of age-related cognitive decline and neurodegenerative diseases. By leveraging advances in biomarker discovery, personalized medicine, and non-pharmacological interventions, researchers are moving closer to realizing the goal of preserving cognitive function and enhancing quality of life for aging populations. Continued investment in research and innovation is essential to address the growing burden of cognitive aging on individuals, families, and society as a whole.

The quest for effective treatments and interventions to combat age-related cognitive decline and neurodegenerative diseases stands as a paramount challenge in contemporary healthcare and biomedical research. Delving into the realms of ongoing investigations into brain aging, we unearth profound implications that could shape the landscape of future therapies and interventions.

Foremost among these implications is the potential for early detection and intervention in age-related cognitive decline. Recent strides in biomarker discovery and neuroimaging techniques offer a glimmer of hope in identifying individuals susceptible to cognitive impairment even before clinical symptoms manifest. Biomarkers like amyloid-beta and tau protein levels in cerebrospinal fluid, along with imaging markers of brain atrophy and dysfunction, serve as invaluable tools in unraveling the underlying pathology of neurodegenerative diseases. This early detection paves the way for timely interventions with disease-modifying therapies or lifestyle adjustments, aimed at preserving cognitive faculties and staving off disease progression.

Moreover, ongoing research casts light on the diverse nature of cognitive aging and dementia, accentuating the necessity for personalized treatment approaches. The pace and severity of cognitive decline vary among older adults, influenced by an interplay of genetics, lifestyle choices, and comorbidities. Personalized medicine endeavors, guided by genetic and biomarker data, strive to tailor treatment regimens to the distinctive needs and attributes of each patient. By honing in on specific disease pathways or risk factors, personalized interventions hold promise for heightened efficacy and diminished side effects, departing from traditional one-size-fits-all methodologies.

Another profound implication emanating from ongoing research is the potential for disease-modifying therapies to arrest or decelerate the progression of neurodegenerative diseases like Alzheimer's and Parkinson's. Despite the prolonged research endeavors, there remains a stark absence of treatments capable of reversing or halting the underlying neurodegenerative processes. Nonetheless, recent insights into disease mechanisms and therapeutic targets kindle optimism for the emergence of novel interventions. Experimental drugs targeting amyloid-beta, tau protein, neuroinflammation, and synaptic dysfunction are currently undergoing clinical trials, with preliminary findings evoking optimism. Concurrently, investigations into gene therapies, stem cell-based approaches, and neuroprotective agents hold promise as potential game-changers in the realm of neurodegenerative disease treatment.

Beyond pharmacological avenues, lifestyle modifications and non-pharmacological interventions harbor the potential to mitigate cognitive decline and bolster brain health in aging populations. A panoply of interventions encompassing physical exercise, cognitive training, social engagement, and dietary adjustments have demonstrated favorable impacts on cognitive function, potentially reducing the risk of dementia. The advent of digital health technologies, including smartphone applications, wearable devices, and telemedicine platforms, heralds scalable and cost-effective solutions for delivering personalized interventions and remotely monitoring cognitive health.

Further fueling optimism, ongoing investigations into the gut-brain axis and the role of the microbiome in cognitive aging offer tantalizing prospects for novel therapeutic strategies. Explorations into prebiotics, probiotics, and fecal microbiota transplantation as potential modulators of the gut microbiota present promising avenues for enhancing cognitive function in older adults. Additionally, targeting inflammation and oxidative stress pathways through dietary supplements or nutraceuticals could confer neuroprotective benefits and bolster resilience against age-related cognitive decline.

In the pursuit of translating research findings into tangible clinical benefits, collaboration stands as an indispensable cornerstone. Multifaceted alliances between academia, industry, and government agencies facilitate the development of groundbreaking therapies, biomarkers, and diagnostic tools for neurodegenerative diseases. Regulatory oversight ensures the safety and efficacy of emerging treatments, while healthcare providers and patient advocacy organizations play pivotal roles in disseminating awareness and facilitating access to care for individuals grappling with cognitive aging and dementia.

In summation, the ongoing research endeavors in brain aging portend a paradigm shift in the diagnosis, treatment, and management of age-related cognitive decline and neurodegenerative diseases. Through harnessing advances in biomarker discovery, personalized medicine, and non-pharmacological interventions, researchers inch closer to the overarching goal of preserving cognitive vitality and enhancing the quality of life for aging populations. Sustained investments in research and innovation emerge as imperatives in tackling the burgeoning burden of cognitive aging, resonating across individuals, families, and society at large.

Upon these foundational pillars, it becomes evident that the journey towards combating age-related cognitive decline is multifaceted and dynamic. Central to this endeavor is the imperative to elucidate the intricate interplay between genetic predispositions and environmental factors in shaping cognitive trajectories. By unraveling the genetic underpinnings of cognitive aging through genome-wide association studies (GWAS) and other molecular approaches, researchers aim to identify novel therapeutic targets and prognostic markers that could revolutionize personalized interventions.

Moreover, the advent of cutting-edge technologies such as artificial intelligence (AI) and machine learning holds immense promise in enhancing our understanding of complex neurodegenerative diseases. These computational approaches enable the analysis of vast datasets encompassing genomics, proteomics, and neuroimaging, thereby unraveling intricate disease mechanisms and uncovering hidden patterns. By leveraging AI-driven algorithms, researchers can accelerate the discovery of novel biomarkers, identify optimal treatment regimens, and predict disease progression with unprecedented accuracy.

Furthermore, the integration of interdisciplinary perspectives is paramount in driving innovation and fostering synergies across disparate fields. Collaborations between neuroscientists, clinicians, computer scientists, and engineers facilitate the development of novel diagnostic tools, therapeutic modalities, and assistive technologies for individuals with cognitive impairments. The convergence of neuroscience with disciplines such as robotics and nanotechnology opens new frontiers in the realm of neurorehabilitation, offering hope for restoring lost cognitive functions and improving quality of life.

In tandem with these scientific endeavors, there is a growing recognition of the pivotal role played by societal factors in shaping cognitive aging trajectories. Socioeconomic disparities, educational attainment, access to healthcare, and environmental factors exert profound influences on cognitive health outcomes, underscoring the importance of adopting a holistic approach to cognitive aging research. Initiatives aimed at promoting lifelong learning, social inclusion, and equitable access to healthcare services hold promise in mitigating cognitive disparities and fostering cognitive resilience across diverse populations.

Moreover, fostering a culture of cognitive health promotion and awareness is essential in empowering individuals to take proactive steps towards preserving cognitive vitality. Public health campaigns, community-based interventions, and educational initiatives play pivotal roles in disseminating evidence-based strategies for brain health maintenance and cognitive resilience. By raising awareness about modifiable risk factors such as sedentary lifestyles, poor nutrition, and social isolation, individuals can make informed lifestyle choices that promote cognitive well-being and mitigate the risk of neurodegenerative diseases.

Furthermore, addressing the unique needs of vulnerable populations, including older adults from underserved communities and individuals with cognitive disabilities, necessitates a concerted effort to promote inclusivity and accessibility in healthcare delivery. Culturally sensitive interventions, caregiver support programs, and innovative telehealth solutions tailored to the needs of diverse populations are imperative in bridging the gap in cognitive healthcare disparities and ensuring equitable access to diagnostic and therapeutic services.

The pursuit of effective treatments and interventions for age-related cognitive decline and neurodegenerative diseases demands a comprehensive and collaborative approach that transcends disciplinary boundaries and addresses the complex interplay of biological, social, and environmental factors. By harnessing the power of scientific innovation, technological advancement, and societal engagement, we can aspire to transform the trajectory of cognitive aging, ushering in an era of enhanced cognitive resilience, improved quality of life, and equitable access to cognitive healthcare for all.

Furthermore, as we delve deeper into the complexities of age-related cognitive decline, it becomes evident that the intersectionality of health disparities and cognitive aging presents unique challenges that necessitate tailored interventions. Individuals from marginalized communities, including racial and ethnic minorities, LGBTQ+ individuals, and those with limited socioeconomic resources, often face disproportionate burdens of cognitive decline due to systemic inequities in healthcare access, education, and social support. Addressing these disparities requires a multifaceted approach that acknowledges the intersecting influences of race, ethnicity, gender identity, sexual orientation, socioeconomic status, and other social determinants of health on cognitive aging trajectories.

In addition, the role of psychological and emotional well-being in cognitive health cannot be overstated. Chronic stress, depression, anxiety, and other mental health conditions have been linked to accelerated cognitive decline and increased risk of neurodegenerative diseases. Interventions aimed at promoting mental resilience, stress management, and emotional support are integral components of comprehensive strategies for preserving cognitive function and enhancing overall well-being in aging populations. Mindfulness-based interventions, cognitive-behavioral therapy, and social support networks offer promising avenues for bolstering mental health and resilience against cognitive decline.

Moreover, fostering an age-friendly environment that promotes cognitive engagement, social connectivity, and meaningful participation in community life is essential for optimizing cognitive health outcomes across the lifespan. Age-friendly cities and communities initiatives advocate for urban planning, infrastructure development, and social policies that accommodate the needs of older adults, including accessible public spaces, transportation options, housing facilities, and recreational opportunities. By creating environments that support active aging and social inclusion, communities can enhance the cognitive vitality and quality of life for individuals of all ages.

Additionally, the role of caregivers and support networks in the care and management of individuals with cognitive impairments cannot be understated. Family caregivers, healthcare professionals, and community organizations play vital roles in providing assistance, advocacy, and emotional support to individuals with cognitive decline and their families. Respite care programs, caregiver training, and support groups offer much-needed resources and respite to caregivers, mitigating caregiver burden and promoting the well-being of both caregivers and care recipients.

Furthermore, fostering a culture of lifelong learning and cognitive stimulation is paramount in maintaining cognitive vitality and resilience across the lifespan. Educational initiatives, cognitive enrichment programs, and lifelong learning opportunities offer avenues for intellectual growth, skill development, and cognitive engagement at every stage of life. By encouraging curiosity, creativity, and continued learning, individuals can enhance cognitive reserve and mitigate the risk of cognitive decline as they age.

Addressing the multifaceted challenges of age-related cognitive decline requires a comprehensive and inclusive approach that encompasses biological, psychological, social, and environmental factors. By fostering collaborative partnerships, promoting health equity, and advocating for age-friendly policies and environments, we can work towards creating a future where cognitive aging is characterized by resilience, empowerment, and dignity for individuals of all backgrounds and abilities. Through collective action and shared commitment, we can aspire to build a society where cognitive health is valued, protected, and prioritized as a fundamental human right.

Chapter VII. Conclusion

Recap of key points discussed in the book

Understanding the essence of a book encompasses more than just its narrative or storyline. It delves into the core messages, insights, and revelations it imparts. When it comes to summarizing a book, particularly one that tackles complex themes such as aging and memory, distilling its key points is paramount. In exploring the profound topic of aging and memory, the journey within the pages of such a book unfolds like a tapestry woven with scientific discoveries, personal anecdotes, and philosophical reflections.

The essence of aging and memory often revolves around the intricate dance between biological processes and environmental influences. Throughout the book, readers are taken on a captivating voyage through the labyrinth of neurobiology, psychology, and sociology, unraveling the mysteries that shroud the aging mind. From the physiological changes in the brain's structure to the psychological adaptations in memory formation, every chapter unfurls a new layer of understanding.

One of the central themes that emerge from the book is the plasticity of the aging brain. Contrary to the long-held belief that cognitive decline is an inevitable aspect of aging, the narrative challenges readers to rethink their perceptions. Through compelling research findings and real-life examples, the book illuminates the remarkable resilience of the aging brain. It underscores the importance of nurturing cognitive vitality through lifelong learning, mental exercises, and social engagement.

Moreover, the book delves into the multifaceted nature of memory and its intricacies. It explores the nuances between different types of memory, from episodic recollections to procedural know-how. By dissecting the mechanisms underlying memory formation and retrieval, readers gain a deeper appreciation for the complexities of human cognition. Furthermore, the book sheds light on the phenomenon of forgetting, portraying it not as a flaw but as an integral part of the memory system.

In essence, the key points discussed in the book converge to form a holistic understanding of aging and memory. It challenges prevailing stereotypes and offers a nuanced perspective that celebrates the resilience and adaptability of the aging mind. By synthesizing scientific knowledge with personal insights, the book enriches readers' understanding of what it means to age gracefully and mindfully.

Aging and memory, as explored within the pages of this book, intricately blend biological processes with environmental influences. Readers embark on a captivating journey through neurobiology, psychology, and sociology, unraveling the mysteries surrounding the aging mind. Each chapter peels back another layer, revealing the physiological changes in brain structure and the psychological adaptations in memory formation.

A central theme emerges: the plasticity of the aging brain. Contrary to the belief that cognitive decline is inevitable with age, these narratives challenge readers to reconsider. Backed by compelling research and real-life examples, they showcase the remarkable resilience of the aging brain. The importance of nurturing cognitive vitality through lifelong learning, mental exercises, and social engagement is underscored.

Furthermore, the complexity of memory is explored. Different types of memory, from episodic recollections to procedural know-how, are examined in detail. By dissecting the mechanisms of memory formation and retrieval, readers gain a deeper understanding of human cognition. The book also reframes forgetting, presenting it not as a flaw but as an integral aspect of the memory system.

In essence, the book offers a holistic understanding of aging and memory. It challenges stereotypes and celebrates the resilience of the aging mind. By synthesizing scientific knowledge with personal insights, it enriches readers' understanding of aging gracefully and mindfully.

Further exploration of the book reveals intricate layers of understanding regarding aging and memory. It goes beyond mere acknowledgment of cognitive decline in old age to highlight the potential for growth and adaptation. Through detailed analysis, readers come to appreciate the dynamic interplay between biological, psychological, and social factors in shaping cognitive function over time.

The narrative doesn't shy away from the complexities inherent in the aging process. It acknowledges the challenges and limitations that individuals may face as they grow older while emphasizing the capacity for resilience and adaptation. By presenting a balanced view of aging, the book encourages readers to approach the subject with nuance and empathy, fostering a deeper understanding of the aging experience.

Moreover, the book delves into the impact of lifestyle choices and environmental factors on cognitive health. It emphasizes the importance of maintaining a healthy lifestyle, including regular exercise, balanced nutrition, and adequate sleep, in promoting cognitive function as people age. Additionally, the role of social connections and meaningful activities in supporting cognitive well-being is highlighted, underscoring the importance of holistic approaches to healthy aging.

Furthermore, the book addresses the ethical considerations surrounding aging and memory care. It raises important questions about autonomy, dignity, and quality of life for older adults, prompting readers to reflect on their own attitudes and beliefs towards aging and end-of-life care. By engaging with these complex ethical issues, the book encourages readers to approach aging with compassion and empathy, fostering a more inclusive and age-friendly society.

Upon the multifaceted nature of aging and memory, the book delves into the impact of cultural and societal attitudes on perceptions of aging. It examines how ageism, discrimination, and stereotypes can influence the way individuals view themselves and others as they grow older. By shedding light on these societal influences, the book encourages readers to challenge ageist beliefs and advocate for a more inclusive and equitable society for people of all ages.

Additionally, the book explores the role of technology in supporting cognitive health and memory function in older adults. It discusses the potential benefits of digital tools, such as brain training apps and virtual reality simulations, in promoting cognitive stimulation and engagement. However, it also raises important considerations about accessibility, privacy, and digital literacy, highlighting the need for thoughtful and ethical use of technology in aging and memory care.

Furthermore, the book examines the intersectionality of aging, considering how factors such as gender, race, ethnicity, socioeconomic status, and sexual orientation can intersect to shape individuals' experiences of aging and memory loss. It emphasizes the importance of recognizing and addressing these intersecting identities in research, policy, and practice to ensure equitable access to resources and support for all older adults.

Moreover, the book examines the role of caregiving in the context of aging and memory loss. It explores the challenges and rewards of caring for aging loved ones, highlighting the importance of compassion, patience, and self-care for caregivers. By sharing practical tips and resources, the book aims to empower caregivers to navigate the caregiving journey with confidence and resilience, promoting positive outcomes for both caregivers and care recipients.

The book offers a rich and nuanced exploration of aging and memory that encompasses scientific, cultural, ethical, and emotional dimensions. It challenges readers to reconsider their assumptions about aging and encourages them to approach the aging process with curiosity, compassion, and empathy. By fostering a deeper understanding of aging and memory, the book empowers readers to embrace the complexities of later life with grace and resilience.

As an exploration, the book delves into the impact of socioeconomic disparities on aging and memory outcomes. It examines how factors such as access to healthcare, education, and financial resources can shape individuals' cognitive health trajectories as they age. By highlighting the disproportionate burden of cognitive decline experienced by marginalized communities, the book calls attention to the urgent need for equitable policies and interventions to address health disparities and promote cognitive well-being for all.

Furthermore, the book investigates the role of lifelong learning and intellectual engagement in supporting cognitive vitality throughout the aging process. It explores how activities such as reading, learning new skills, and engaging in intellectually stimulating hobbies can help preserve cognitive function and promote brain health in later life. By emphasizing the importance of lifelong learning, the book inspires readers to cultivate a curious and intellectually active lifestyle that fosters resilience and cognitive flourishing.

In addition, the book examines the impact of environmental factors, such as urban design and community infrastructure, on aging and memory outcomes. It discusses how age-friendly environments that prioritize accessibility, walkability, and social connectivity can promote healthy aging and support cognitive well-being for older adults. By advocating for age-friendly policies and urban planning initiatives, the book seeks to create environments that empower older adults to live independently, actively, and meaningfully in their communities.

Moreover, the book explores the concept of successful aging and its implications for understanding aging and memory. It challenges traditional biomedical models of aging by emphasizing the importance of holistic approaches that encompass physical, cognitive, emotional, and social dimensions of well-being. By reframing aging as a dynamic and multifaceted process that encompasses growth, adaptation, and resilience, the book offers a more optimistic and empowering perspective on aging that celebrates the strengths and capabilities of older adults.

The book examines the role of advocacy and activism in promoting social change and advancing the rights and dignity of older adults. It highlights the importance of collective action and community engagement in challenging ageism, advocating for age-friendly policies, and fostering inclusive communities that value and support people of all ages. By empowering readers to become agents of continuing the discourse, the book delves into the evolving field of gerontology and its implications for understanding aging and memory. It explores how interdisciplinary research and innovative methodologies are reshaping our understanding of aging and memory, from the molecular mechanisms of neurodegeneration to the societal dynamics of aging populations. By highlighting the cutting-edge research and emerging trends in the field, the book provides readers with a glimpse into the future of aging research and its potential impact on society.

Furthermore, the book examines the role of resilience and coping strategies in mitigating the impact of age-related changes on memory and cognitive function. It discusses how factors such as personality traits, coping mechanisms, and social support networks can influence individuals' ability to adapt to age-related challenges and maintain cognitive well-being. By emphasizing the importance of resilience-building interventions and supportive environments, the book offers practical guidance for promoting positive aging outcomes and enhancing quality of life for older adults.

In addition, the book explores the intersections between aging, memory, and creativity. It discusses how creativity can serve as a powerful tool for self-expression, personal growth, and cognitive enrichment in later life. By showcasing examples of older adults who have embraced creativity as a means of coping with age-related changes and finding purpose and fulfillment, the book challenges stereotypes about aging and celebrates the potential for creativity to flourish across the lifespan.

Moreover, the book examines the role of spirituality and existential meaning-making in shaping individuals' experiences of aging and memory. It explores how concepts such as purpose, transcendence, and connectedness can provide a sense of meaning and resilience in the face of age-related challenges and transitions. By integrating insights from spirituality and existential psychology into discussions of aging and memory, the book offers a holistic framework for understanding the deeper dimensions of the aging process and fostering spiritual well-being in later life.

The book considers the global implications of aging and memory loss in an increasingly interconnected world. It examines how demographic shifts, urbanization, and globalization are transforming the landscape of aging and memory care, creating both challenges and opportunities for individuals, families, and societies worldwide. By exploring cross-cultural perspectives on aging and memory, the book highlights the importance of cultural competence, diversity, and inclusion in addressing the needs of aging populations around the globe.

The book offers a nuanced and expansive exploration of aging and memory that spans disciplines, cultures, and generations. It challenges readers to think critically about the complexities of aging and memory and inspires them to engage with these issues with empathy, curiosity, and creativity. By fostering a deeper understanding of aging and memory, the book empowers readers to navigate the aging process with grace, resilience, and purpose, enriching their lives and the lives of those around them, the book encourages them to work towards a more just, equitable, and age-friendly society for current and future generations.

The book offers a comprehensive and multidimensional exploration of aging and memory that encompasses scientific, social, cultural, and ethical perspectives. It challenges readers to reconsider their assumptions about aging and memory and inspires them to take action to promote cognitive well-being, social justice, and inclusivity for people of all ages. By fostering a deeper understanding of aging and memory, the book empowers readers to embrace aging with resilience, dignity, and purpose, creating a brighter future for individuals and communities alike.

Call to action for readers to prioritize brain health and aging

As we traverse the labyrinth of life, our cognitive well-being emerges as a precious gem that requires nurturing and safeguarding. In an era dominated by the frenetic pace of modern living, it's easy to overlook the profound importance of brain health and aging. Yet, amidst the hustle and bustle of daily existence, our cognitive vitality stands as a cornerstone of our overall well-being.

The call to action for readers to prioritize brain health and aging transcends mere rhetoric; it embodies a fundamental shift in mindset and lifestyle. It beckons individuals to embark on a journey of self-discovery and empowerment, championing the principles of proactive health management and holistic well-being. At its core, this call to action implores individuals to become stewards of their cognitive destiny, embracing a proactive approach to brain health.

Central to this call to action is the recognition that aging is not a static process but a dynamic continuum characterized by ongoing growth and adaptation. Rather than succumbing to the myths of cognitive decline and senescence, readers are encouraged to cultivate a mindset of resilience and empowerment. By embracing lifestyle practices that foster cognitive vitality, such as regular exercise, healthy nutrition, mental stimulation, and social engagement, individuals can fortify their cognitive reserves and mitigate the risk of age-related decline.

Moreover, the call to action emphasizes the importance of fostering a supportive environment that champions brain health and aging across all facets of society. From policymakers and healthcare providers to educators and caregivers, there exists a collective responsibility to prioritize initiatives that promote cognitive well-being and aging-in-place. By fostering a culture of lifelong learning, age-friendly communities, and accessible healthcare services, we can empower individuals of all ages to thrive and flourish.

Ultimately, the call to action for readers to prioritize brain health and aging is rooted in the belief that each individual possesses the agency to shape their cognitive destiny. By embracing the principles of proactive health management, lifelong learning, and social connectedness, individuals can embark on a journey of cognitive flourishing that transcends the boundaries of age. As stewards of our cognitive well-being, let us heed this call to action with steadfast resolve, knowing that the choices we make today will shape the cognitive landscapes of tomorrow.

In the intricate web of life's journey, the preservation of our cognitive well-being emerges as a treasure worthy of diligent care and protection. In a world marked by the relentless hustle of contemporary living, it's all too easy to underestimate the profound significance of brain health and its correlation with the aging process. Nevertheless, amidst the ceaseless commotion of our daily routines, the vitality of our cognitive faculties remains a pivotal pillar of our overall welfare.

Encouraging readers to prioritize brain health and aging extends beyond mere words; it embodies a profound shift in perspective and lifestyle. It invites individuals to embark on a voyage of self-discovery and empowerment, advocating for the principles of proactive health management and holistic well-being. At its essence, this call to action urges individuals to assume responsibility for their cognitive fate, embracing a proactive stance towards the preservation of brain health.

At the heart of this call to action lies the acknowledgment that aging is not a stationary state but rather a dynamic process characterized by continuous evolution and adaptation. Instead of succumbing to the misconceptions surrounding cognitive decline and senescence, readers are urged to cultivate a mindset of resilience and self-empowerment. Through the adoption of lifestyle practices conducive to cognitive vitality, such as regular physical activity, balanced nutrition, mental engagement, and meaningful social interactions, individuals can bolster their cognitive reserves and mitigate the risks associated with age-related deterioration.

Furthermore, the call to action underscores the significance of nurturing a supportive milieu that advocates for brain health and aging across all sectors of society. From policymakers and healthcare professionals to educators and caregivers, there exists a collective obligation to prioritize endeavors aimed at promoting cognitive well-being and enabling individuals to age gracefully within their communities. By fostering environments conducive to lifelong learning, cultivating age-friendly communities, and ensuring equitable access to healthcare services, we can empower individuals of all ages to lead fulfilling and enriching lives.

In the intricate tapestry of human existence, the preservation of cognitive well-being emerges as a cornerstone essential for navigating life's labyrinthine paths. Amidst the cacophony of modern living, where every moment seems filled with haste and distraction, the value of nurturing and safeguarding brain health and aging often gets obscured. However, within this frenetic pace, the importance of maintaining cognitive vitality remains a vital component of our overall wellness, deserving of deliberate attention and care.

Encouraging readers to prioritize brain health and aging transcends mere suggestion; it necessitates a profound paradigm shift in how we perceive and approach our well-being. It calls upon individuals to embark on a transformative journey of self-discovery and empowerment, championing the principles of proactive health management and holistic flourishing. At its core, this call to action urges us to assume an active role in shaping our cognitive destinies, embracing a mindset that prioritizes the preservation and enhancement of brain function throughout the aging process.

In the intricate dance of life's complexities, the preservation of cognitive well-being emerges as a non-negotiable aspect that demands our utmost attention and care. In a world where the relentless pace of modernity often obscures the significance of mental health and aging, it becomes imperative to shine a spotlight on the importance of nurturing our cognitive faculties. Amidst the chaos and clamor of daily existence, our cognitive vitality serves as a compass guiding us towards holistic well-being and fulfillment.

At the heart of this call to action lies the understanding that aging is not a one-dimensional process but rather a multifaceted journey marked by growth, adaptation, and resilience. Instead of passively accepting the narrative of cognitive decline, we are urged to embrace the concept of neuroplasticity—the brain's remarkable ability to reorganize and adapt in response to experiences. By engaging in activities that stimulate neural pathways, such as learning new skills, exploring novel experiences, and practicing mindfulness, individuals can harness the brain's inherent capacity for regeneration and renewal.

Moreover, the call to action emphasizes the need for societal support systems that champion brain health and aging across diverse domains. From implementing policies that promote age-friendly communities to ensuring equitable access to healthcare services and educational resources, there exists a collective responsibility to create environments that nurture cognitive well-being. By fostering a culture of inclusivity, compassion, and respect for individuals of all ages, we can create a society where cognitive flourishing is viewed as a shared priority.

In the grand tapestry of human existence, the preservation of cognitive well-being emerges as a fundamental thread weaving through the fabric of our lives. In a fast-paced world where the pursuit of productivity often takes precedence over self-care, it becomes imperative to recognize the intrinsic value of nurturing our cognitive health. Amidst the noise and distractions of modern living, our cognitive faculties serve as the foundation upon which we build our experiences, relationships, and sense of identity.

Encouraging readers to prioritize brain health and aging requires a paradigm shift—a reevaluation of our values and priorities in the pursuit of a balanced and fulfilling life. It invites individuals to embark on a journey of self-discovery and empowerment, where the cultivation of cognitive resilience becomes a guiding principle. At its core, this call to action urges us to embrace a holistic approach to health, one that encompasses not only physical well-being but also mental, emotional, and social aspects of our lives.

At the heart of this call to action lies the recognition that aging is a natural and inevitable part of the human experience, yet it need not be synonymous with cognitive decline. Instead of viewing aging as a decline towards obsolescence, we can reframe it as an opportunity for growth, wisdom, and continued self-actualization. By embracing the concept of "active aging," individuals can adopt lifestyle habits and attitudes that promote cognitive vitality and resilience throughout the lifespan.

Moreover, the call to action extends beyond the individual level to encompass broader societal changes that foster environments conducive to cognitive well-being. From creating age-friendly communities that support active living and social engagement to implementing policies that prioritize access to healthcare and educational resources for older adults, there is a collective responsibility to ensure that individuals can age with dignity and purpose. By investing in initiatives that promote lifelong learning, intergenerational connections, and inclusive healthcare practices, we can build a society where cognitive flourishing is valued and accessible to all.

Final thoughts on the importance of understanding the brain science behind aging and forgetting

In the grand tapestry of human existence, the journey of aging and forgetting emerges as a poignant reflection of our shared humanity. It is a journey marked by the passage of time, the ebb and flow of memories, and the inexorable march of cognitive change. Yet, amidst the complexities and uncertainties that shroud the aging mind, there exists a beacon of hope and understanding: the illuminating insights of brain science.

The importance of understanding the brain science behind aging and forgetting cannot be overstated. It serves as a guiding light amidst the labyrinthine depths of cognitive decline, offering clarity, empowerment, and a sense of purpose. By unraveling the mysteries that shroud the aging brain, we gain invaluable insights into the underlying mechanisms of memory formation, retention, and retrieval.

One of the most profound realizations gleaned from the study of brain science is the remarkable plasticity of the aging brain. Contrary to the long-held belief that cognitive decline is an inevitable aspect of aging, research has shown that the brain retains a remarkable capacity for growth and adaptation throughout the lifespan. This realization underscores the transformative potential of lifestyle interventions, cognitive training, and social engagement in preserving cognitive vitality and mitigating the risk of age-related decline.

Furthermore, understanding the brain science behind aging and forgetting offers profound implications for the development of novel therapeutic interventions and preventive strategies. From pharmacological interventions targeting neurodegenerative diseases to lifestyle interventions promoting cognitive resilience, the insights gleaned from brain science hold the promise of enhancing the quality of life for individuals across the aging spectrum.

Moreover, by shedding light on the phenomenon of forgetting, brain science challenges prevailing misconceptions and stigmas surrounding memory loss and cognitive decline. Rather than viewing forgetting as a sign of weakness or incompetence, we come to understand it as a natural and adaptive process inherent to the functioning of the memory system. This reframing empowers individuals to embrace the complexities of memory and aging with grace, resilience, and self-compassion.

The importance of understanding the brain science behind aging and forgetting cannot be understated. It offers a beacon of hope amidst the uncertainties of cognitive change, empowering individuals to navigate the journey of aging with resilience, dignity, and purpose. As we stand on the precipice of a new era in brain health and aging, let us embrace the transformative potential of brain science to shape a future where cognitive vitality knows no bounds.

In the vast expanse of human experience, the process of aging and the accompanying phenomenon of forgetting stand out as poignant reminders of our shared humanity. These aspects of life are characterized by the passage of time, the fluctuation of memories, and the inevitable shifts in cognitive abilities. However, amidst the complexities that surround aging minds, there exists a glimmer of hope: the illuminating insights provided by brain science.

Understanding the intricacies of brain science in relation to aging and forgetting holds immense importance. It serves as a guiding beacon in the maze of cognitive decline, offering clarity, empowerment, and a renewed sense of purpose. Through delving into the mysteries of the aging brain, we gain invaluable knowledge about how memories form, persist, and sometimes fade away.

Perhaps one of the most profound revelations from the realm of brain science is the remarkable plasticity of the aging brain. Contrary to long-held assumptions, research has shown that the brain possesses an extraordinary ability to adapt and grow throughout life. This understanding highlights the potential for lifestyle changes, cognitive exercises, and social interactions to bolster cognitive functions and mitigate the effects of aging.

Moreover, comprehending the brain's mechanisms in aging and forgetting holds significant promise for developing new therapeutic approaches and preventative measures. Whether through medications targeting neurodegenerative conditions or interventions aimed at promoting cognitive resilience, insights from brain science offer hope for enhancing the well-being of individuals as they age.

Furthermore, by shedding light on the processes of forgetting, brain science challenges societal misconceptions and stigmas surrounding memory loss. Rather than viewing forgetfulness as a flaw, it is recognized as a natural aspect of memory function. This shift in perspective empowers individuals to embrace the complexities of memory and aging with acceptance and self-compassion.

Moreover, the insights gleaned from brain science offer profound implications for society as a whole. By understanding the processes of aging and forgetting at a neurological level, we can develop more compassionate and effective support systems for individuals experiencing cognitive decline. This includes tailored care plans, educational initiatives, and policies that prioritize brain health across the lifespan.

Furthermore, the application of brain science in the realm of aging and forgetting extends to areas beyond individual health. It has implications for workforce development, as businesses and organizations adapt to accommodate an aging workforce by implementing strategies that support cognitive wellness. Additionally, urban planning and design can be informed by research on brain health to create environments that promote active lifestyles and social connections, which are vital for maintaining cognitive vitality as we age.

Importantly, the integration of brain science into public discourse on aging and forgetting fosters greater awareness and understanding. This can help dispel myths and misconceptions, reducing the stigma associated with cognitive decline and memory loss. By fostering open conversations, we create a more inclusive society where individuals feel supported and empowered to seek help when needed.

Furthermore, ongoing research in the field of brain science continues to uncover new insights into the complexities of aging and forgetting. Advances in technology, such as neuroimaging techniques and big data analysis, provide researchers with unprecedented tools to study the brain in unprecedented detail. These advancements hold the potential to unlock even deeper understanding of the mechanisms underlying cognitive aging, leading to more targeted interventions and personalized treatments in the future.

Additionally, the interdisciplinary nature of brain science fosters collaboration across diverse fields, from psychology and neuroscience to medicine and public health. By bringing together experts with varied perspectives and expertise, we can tackle the complex challenges posed by aging and forgetting more effectively. This collaborative approach not only accelerates scientific progress but also ensures that research findings are translated into practical solutions that benefit individuals and communities worldwide.

In essence, the journey of aging and forgetting is one that touches us all, transcending cultural, geographical, and socioeconomic boundaries. By embracing the insights offered by brain science, we can navigate this journey with greater understanding, compassion, and resilience. As we continue to unravel the mysteries of the aging brain, let us remain committed to harnessing the transformative power of knowledge to create a world where every individual can age with dignity, grace, and cognitive vitality.

Moreover, the impact of brain science on aging and forgetting extends to the realm of education and lifelong learning. By understanding how the brain changes over time, educators can develop more effective teaching methods that cater to the needs of older adults. This includes implementing strategies to enhance memory retention, promote cognitive flexibility, and facilitate continuous intellectual stimulation. Lifelong learning programs can also be tailored to capitalize on the brain's plasticity, offering opportunities for personal growth and cognitive enrichment throughout adulthood.

Furthermore, the insights from brain science underscore the importance of holistic approaches to health and well-being as we age. Physical exercise, nutrition, sleep, and stress management all play crucial roles in maintaining brain health and cognitive function. By adopting healthy lifestyle habits, individuals can optimize their brain health and reduce the risk of age-related cognitive decline. Public health initiatives aimed at promoting brain-healthy behaviors can have far-reaching benefits for individuals, families, and communities.

In addition, the application of brain science in aging and forgetting has implications for the field of gerontology and geriatrics. Healthcare professionals can utilize neurocognitive assessments and biomarkers to detect early signs of cognitive impairment and intervene proactively. Moreover, personalized medicine approaches based on individual differences in brain structure and function hold promise for tailoring treatments to each person's unique needs and preferences.

Furthermore, the insights gained from brain science can inform policy decisions aimed at addressing the challenges of an aging population. Governments and policymakers can use evidence-based approaches to develop comprehensive aging policies that support healthy aging, promote social inclusion, and provide equitable access to healthcare and support services. By investing in research, education, and infrastructure, societies can create environments that enable older adults to age with dignity and independence.

Additionally, the ethical implications of brain science in aging and forgetting warrant careful consideration. As technologies advance and our understanding of the brain deepens, questions arise about issues such as cognitive enhancement, end-of-life decision-making, and the preservation of personal identity in the face of cognitive decline. Ethical frameworks and guidelines can help navigate these complex issues, ensuring that advancements in brain science are used responsibly and ethically to benefit individuals and society as a whole.

The intersection of brain science with aging and forgetting represents a frontier of knowledge with profound implications for individuals, communities, and societies worldwide. By harnessing the insights provided by brain science, we can revolutionize how we perceive and address the challenges of aging, memory loss, and cognitive decline. Through interdisciplinary collaboration, holistic approaches to health and well-being, and ethical consideration of emerging technologies, we can pave the way for a future where aging is embraced as a natural part of the human experience, and where every individual can age with dignity, purpose, and cognitive vitality.

Furthermore, the integration of brain science into cultural narratives and creative expressions can foster greater awareness and empathy towards individuals experiencing aging and memory loss. Literature, film, art, and other forms of media can serve as powerful vehicles for storytelling that humanize the experiences of older adults and challenge stereotypes associated with aging and forgetfulness. By highlighting the richness and complexity of these experiences, creative works can spark meaningful conversations and inspire societal change.

Moreover, the role of social support networks in promoting brain health and resilience cannot be overstated. Strong social connections have been linked to better cognitive function, reduced risk of dementia, and increased longevity. Community-based initiatives that foster social engagement, intergenerational interactions, and peer support can help combat feelings of isolation and loneliness often experienced by older adults. By building inclusive communities that value and support individuals of all ages, we can create environments that promote cognitive well-being and enhance overall quality of life.

In addition, the globalization of aging presents both opportunities and challenges for societies around the world. As populations age and life expectancies increase, diverse cultural perspectives on aging and memory may intersect and influence one another. This cultural exchange can enrich our understanding of aging and memory across different societies and provide valuable insights into universal aspects of the human experience. However, it also requires careful consideration of cultural nuances and context-specific approaches to aging-related issues, including healthcare, social support, and end-of-life care.

Furthermore, the empowerment of older adults as active participants in research and advocacy is essential for driving positive change in the field of aging and memory. By involving older adults in the co-design and implementation of research studies, healthcare interventions, and policy initiatives, we can ensure that their voices and experiences are heard and respected. Similarly, efforts to promote age-friendly environments and policies should prioritize the inclusion of older adults in decision-making processes, allowing them to contribute their expertise and insights to create communities that are supportive and inclusive for people of all ages.

Lastly, the journey of aging and forgetting is not solely an individual experience but also a collective one that shapes the fabric of society. By fostering intergenerational understanding and solidarity, we can bridge the gap between different age groups and create a more cohesive and compassionate society. Intergenerational programs that bring together older adults and younger generations for shared activities, learning opportunities, and mutual support can foster meaningful connections and combat ageism. Through these efforts, we can build a future where individuals of all ages are valued, respected, and supported in their journey of aging and memory.

Additionally, the exploration of spiritual and existential dimensions of aging and memory loss adds depth to our understanding of these phenomena. Many individuals find solace and meaning in spiritual practices, beliefs, and rituals as they navigate the challenges of aging and confront the prospect of memory decline. Spiritual care providers, chaplains, and counselors play important roles in supporting older adults as they grapple with existential questions and seek comfort in their spiritual beliefs. By acknowledging and honoring the spiritual dimensions of aging, we can provide holistic care that addresses the diverse needs of older adults at the end of life and throughout their journey of aging.

Furthermore, advancements in assistive technologies hold promise for enhancing the independence and quality of life of older adults with memory loss. From smartphone apps that provide reminders and prompts for daily tasks to wearable devices that monitor vital signs and detect falls, technology offers innovative solutions for supporting aging in place and mitigating the challenges associated with cognitive decline. By investing in research and development of assistive technologies, we can empower older adults to maintain autonomy and dignity as they age and continue to live fulfilling lives in their own homes and communities.

Moreover, the impact of environmental factors on cognitive health and aging cannot be overlooked. Access to safe and affordable housing, green spaces, and transportation options can significantly influence the well-being of older adults and their ability to remain active and engaged in their communities. Urban planning and design strategies that prioritize age-friendly features, such as walkable neighborhoods, accessible public spaces, and affordable housing options, can create environments that promote healthy aging and enhance the quality of life for people of all ages.

In addition, the recognition of the intersectionality of aging and memory loss is essential for addressing the unique needs and experiences of diverse populations. Older adults from marginalized communities, including racial and ethnic minorities, LGBTQ+ individuals, and people with disabilities, may face compounded barriers to accessing healthcare, social support, and resources for aging well. Efforts to promote health equity and social justice in aging-related policies and programs must consider the intersecting factors of race, ethnicity, gender, sexuality, disability, and socioeconomic status to ensure that all older adults have the opportunity to age with dignity, respect, and equitable access to resources and services.

Lastly, fostering a culture of lifelong learning and curiosity is essential for promoting brain health and cognitive vitality across the lifespan. Opportunities for continued education, intellectual stimulation, and creative expression can help older adults maintain cognitive function, build resilience, and cultivate a sense of purpose and fulfillment in their later years. By embracing a growth mindset and staying intellectually engaged, individuals can continue to learn, grow, and thrive as they age, enriching their lives and contributing to their communities in meaningful ways.

Chapter VIII – The Gut-Brain Axis, the Vagal Nerve, and the Second Brain

Introduction

The gut-brain axis is an intricate system that connects the gastrointestinal tract (GI tract) with the central nervous system (CNS). This bidirectional communication network is crucial for maintaining homeostasis and regulating a wide range of physiological processes, including digestion, immune response, and even mood and behavior. Central to this axis is the vagus nerve, a critical component of the parasympathetic nervous system, which plays a pivotal role in conveying information between the gut and the brain. The concept of the stomach as a "second brain" underscores the complexity and significance of this relationship, highlighting the gut's ability to influence mental states and overall health.

The Anatomy and Physiology of the Gut-Brain Axis

The Enteric Nervous System

The enteric nervous system (ENS), often referred to as the "second brain," is a vast network of neurons embedded in the walls of the gastrointestinal tract. It consists of two major plexuses: the myenteric plexus (Auerbach's plexus), which lies between the longitudinal and circular muscle layers, and the submucosal plexus (Meissner's plexus), located in the submucosa. The ENS contains around 100 million neurons, comparable to the number in the spinal cord, and can function independently of the CNS.

The Vagus Nerve

The vagus nerve, or cranial nerve X, is a primary conduit of information between the gut and the brain. It extends from the brainstem through the neck, thorax, and abdomen, innervating various organs, including the heart, lungs, and digestive tract. The vagus nerve's afferent fibers (those carrying sensory information to the brain) outnumber its efferent fibers (those carrying motor commands to the gut) by approximately 9:1, indicating the significance of gut-to-brain communication.

Gut Microbiota and the Brain

The Microbiome

The human gut harbors a complex community of microorganisms, including bacteria, viruses, fungi, and protozoa, collectively known as the gut microbiota. These microbes play crucial roles in digestion, immune function, and the synthesis of vital nutrients. Emerging research suggests that the gut microbiota also has profound effects on brain function and behavior.

Microbiota-Gut-Brain Axis

The microbiota-gut-brain axis refers to the dynamic interactions between the gut microbiota, the gut, and the brain. Microbial metabolites, such as short-chain fatty acids (SCFAs), neurotransmitters, and neuromodulators, can influence brain function and behavior. For instance, certain gut bacteria can produce serotonin, a neurotransmitter that regulates mood, while others can produce gamma-aminobutyric acid (GABA), which has calming effects on the brain.

Mechanisms of Communication

Neural Pathways

The vagus nerve is the primary neural pathway facilitating communication between the gut and the brain. It transmits signals from the gut to the brainstem and subsequently to various brain regions, including the hypothalamus, amygdala, and prefrontal cortex. This pathway is crucial for the regulation of satiety, stress response, and emotional state.

Humoral Pathways

In addition to neural pathways, the gut-brain axis involves humoral communication through the release of hormones and cytokines. The gut releases hormones such as ghrelin, leptin, and peptide YY, which influence appetite, metabolism, and energy balance. Cytokines, which are signaling molecules involved in immune responses, can also affect brain function and behavior.

Microbial Metabolites

Microbial metabolites produced by the gut microbiota, such as SCFAs, indole derivatives, and bile acids, can cross the blood-brain barrier and influence brain function. SCFAs, in particular, have been shown to modulate neuroinflammation, neurogenesis, and neurotransmission.

The Role of the Vagus Nerve

Vagal Tone and Health

Vagal tone, the level of activity of the vagus nerve, is an important indicator of overall health. High vagal tone is associated with better cardiovascular health, reduced inflammation, and improved emotional regulation. Techniques such as deep breathing, meditation, and yoga can enhance vagal tone and promote a state of relaxation and well-being.

Vagus Nerve Stimulation (VNS)

Vagus nerve stimulation (VNS) is a therapeutic technique that involves electrical stimulation of the vagus nerve. It has been used to treat various conditions, including epilepsy, depression, and inflammatory diseases. VNS can modulate neurotransmitter release, reduce inflammation, and improve neuroplasticity.

The Stomach as a Second Brain

Enteric Autonomy

The ENS's ability to function independently of the CNS has led to its characterization as a second brain. It can regulate gastrointestinal motility, secretion, and blood flow autonomously. This autonomy is crucial for the efficient processing of ingested food and the maintenance of gut homeostasis.

Neurotransmitters in the Gut

The gut produces and responds to many of the same neurotransmitters found in the brain, including serotonin, dopamine, and acetylcholine. Approximately 90% of the body's serotonin is produced in the gut, where it regulates motility, secretion, and sensitivity to pain.

Gut-Brain Axis and Mental Health

Stress and the Gut

Stress can significantly impact gut function, leading to conditions such as irritable bowel syndrome (IBS) and inflammatory bowel disease (IBD). The release of stress hormones, such as cortisol, can alter gut motility, permeability, and microbial composition. Conversely, gut inflammation and dysbiosis (microbial imbalance) can affect stress reactivity and mood.

Gut-Brain Axis in Depression and Anxiety

Emerging evidence suggests that the gut-brain axis plays a role in the pathophysiology of depression and anxiety. Alterations in gut microbiota composition have been observed in individuals with these conditions. Probiotics and prebiotics, which modulate gut microbiota, have shown promise in alleviating symptoms of depression and anxiety in some studies.

Therapeutic Implications

Probiotics and Prebiotics

Probiotics are live microorganisms that confer health benefits when consumed in adequate amounts. They can modulate gut microbiota composition and function, enhance gut barrier integrity, and produce bioactive compounds that influence brain function. Prebiotics are non-digestible food components that promote the growth and activity of beneficial gut bacteria.

Diet and the Gut-Brain Axis

Diet plays a crucial role in shaping the gut microbiota and, consequently, the gut-brain axis. Diets rich in fiber, fermented foods, and polyphenols can promote a healthy gut microbiota and enhance gut-brain communication.

Conversely, diets high in processed foods, sugar, and unhealthy fats can disrupt gut microbiota and impair gut-brain interactions.

Conclusion

The gut-brain axis represents a complex and dynamic system that underscores the interconnectedness of the gut and the brain. The vagus nerve plays a pivotal role in this communication network, influencing various physiological and psychological processes. Understanding the gut-brain axis and its components offers promising avenues for therapeutic interventions targeting mental health, gastrointestinal disorders, and overall well-being. The concept of the stomach as a second brain emphasizes the significance of gut health in maintaining holistic health, highlighting the need for further research and clinical applications in this burgeoning field.

Index: